BREASTFEEDING CHALLENGES

How To Overcome Common Nursing Problems

Lucille M. Mills

The content of this publication is intended to provide information on breastfeeding problems. It is presented to encourage and guide nursing mothers. Always consult a physician when you require medical attention.

BREASTFEEDING CHALLENGES – How To Overcome Common Nursing Problems

i

Table of Contents

ii

v

ABOUT THE AUTHOR

Lucille M. Mills is married with four kids. She worked in a maternal-child health clinic. Besides her research, she had personally experienced difficulties breastfeeding her children.

CHAPTER 1

NATURAL NOURISHMENT FOR BABIES

Infant nutrition may be confusing to new parents. However, breastfeeding is an ideal way of giving your newborn a healthy start in life. With advice from health professionals and encouragement from lactation support groups, first-time mothers can provide the best nourishment to their babies. Infant nutrition not only affects the growth and development of newborns, it also influences their health later in life.

Studies have shown that breastfed children are more intelligent than those fed with formula. The outcomes of these researches confirm that breast milk plays a significant role in brain development. Besides, it boosts the immune system of babies. The immunological requirements of infants for the first couple of years after birth depend on breast milk. In addition to the nutrients contained in human milk, antibodies are also present.

Nutritional Value Of Breast Milk

During the first six months of a baby's life, the mother's milk provides the nutrients needed for development and growth. It also protects the newborn against infections. The breast milk is the perfect nutrient mix for babies. In addition to the nutrients and enzymes, it contains antibodies that provide protection against diseases.

The fluid content of human milk is sufficient for the needs of a baby during the first six months. Supplementation with water is not necessary during this period. However, certain conditions like fever, diarrhea or vomiting can cause a baby to become dehydrated. Rehydration with electrolyte solution is crucial if diarrhea occurs.

You can prepare a simple oral rehydration solution by adding a little salt and sugar to water. The production of dark yellow urine in infants with any of the mentioned health problems indicates dehydration. Babies can also become dehydrated in very hot climates.

The unique components of breast milk surpass all baby formulas. The addition of minerals and vitamins to any chemical formulation cannot offer the properties of this natural nourishment. The human milk is rich in lactose, which is a harmless sugar needed by babies. Feeding a baby with food that contains other sugars may be harmful. The intake of sucrose can damage new teeth in infants.

Nutritional Components of Breast milk

The breast milk contains nutrients needed for healthy growth and development of babies. It is a perfect mix of protein, fats, carbohydrate, vitamins and water. The composition of breast milk changes during a feeding and over the lactation period. However, the proportion of the nutrients in breast milk differs from the content of milk obtainable from other mammals. Due to its uniqueness, breast milk is the ideal food for newborns.

Protein

Breast milk contains immunoglobulin A and other proteins that protect infants against bacterial and viral infection. Besides being a major calorie source, the fat found in breast milk is essential for nervous system and brain development. The hindmilk contains more fat than the foremilk which babies get at the beginning of each feeding.

Fats

The fat in breast milk digests quickly due to the presence of the enzyme, lipase, in the milk. These self-digesting fats make human milk ideal food for premature babies whose digestive systems are not well-developed to perform its functions.

Carbohydrate

Lactose is the major carbohydrate in breast milk. It aids the absorption of minerals such as magnesium, calcium, and phosphorus. Lactose reduces the microbial load of disease-causing bacteria in the stomach and favors the growth of harmless bacteria.

Vitamins and minerals

The vitamins are essential to an infant's health. The vitamins in human milk can't be compared with those listed on a formula. Even if they have the same milligrams, the amount available for an infant to use differs in both cases. A mother's vitamin intake determines the types and quantity of vitamins present in her breast milk. Consequently, she needs adequate nutrition to provide the vitamins to her baby. Many healthcare providers and even lactation consultants advise nursing mothers to continue prenatal vitamins.

Breast milk gets nutrients where they are needed in an infant's bloodstream instead of the baby's bowels. The minerals contained in breast milk are readily absorbed. Though the levels of phosphorus, calcium, and iron in breast milk are low, babies can easily absorb them. Conversely, the vitamins added to the formula have low bioavailability. The manufacturers increase their concentrations to make up for their low bioavailability.

However, excess unabsorbed minerals can negatively affect formula-fed infants. Unabsorbed iron allows harmful bacteria to thrive in a baby's gut by hindering the growth of the good bacteria. It can also make the stools of infants to be harder with an unpleasant smell.

Besides the nutrients, other components of breast milk help protect infants from infections. They also support the development of babies' immune system. These non-nutritional components of breast milk include digestive enzymes, antimicrobial factors, growth factors, and hormones.

The composition of human milk changes during feedings and over the lactation period. The change in its lipid content in a day depends on the baby's feeding behavior. It is lower when the breast if full before a feeding than towards its end when the breast is less full.

Benefits of breastfeeding for infants

Breast milk provides all the nutrients required by infants for growth. These nutrients are available in forms that are easily digested than the baby formula. Besides being a cost-effective way to feed your baby, the infant can obtain the following benefits from breastfeeding.

Bonding: Breastfeeding satisfies a baby's need for affection and security. The eye contact and physical closeness create a superior bond between mother and baby. The bonding is beneficial to the development of the infant.

Fights infection: The antibodies contained in breast milk help antibodies to fight off bacteria and viruses. Besides, breast milk reduces the risk of gastroenteritis, urinary tract infections, respiratory tract infections, ear infections, and inflammatory bowel disease.

Unlike formula-fed babies, incidences of cold and pneumonia are reduced among breastfed infants. The babies are likely to have fewer trips to the physician and hospitalizations if they are exclusively breastfed for the first 6 months of life without taking infant formulas.

Protection against allergies: Breastfeeding reduces your baby's risk of having eczema, asthma or allergies. It is better to breastfeed than using infant formula if there is a history of allergies or asthma in your family. Besides, proteins in soy milk and cow milk formulas can trigger an allergic reaction.

Easy to digest: Babies can easily break down breast milk than infant formula. Consequently, breastfed babies may have less stomach upset, constipation, and diarrhea.

Prevention of overweight or obesity: Breastfed babies are less likely to become overweight or obese as they grow. Breastfeeding your baby may help him to put on the right amount of weight. However, you have to understand his "satiety cues" to know when the infant is full. Unlike bottle feeding that allows you to determine the quantity of feed consumed, your baby's behavior will help you to avoid overfeeding.

Possible higher IQ scores: Studies suggest that breastfed infants are smarter than their bottle-fed counterparts later in life. Besides, the fatty acids present in breast milk are regarded as brain boosters.

Prevention of SIDS: Most cases of SIDS involve formula-fed babies indicating that breastfeeding can lower the risk of sudden infant death syndrome (SIDS). However, the connection between breastfeeding and SIDS is unclear.

Research suggests that breast milk protect infants from type 1 diabetes, certain cancers, and spinal meningitis. Through breast milk, a mother can transfer immune factors to her baby. Consequently, breastfed infants show a better antibody response than formula-fed babies, making vaccines more effective.

Breastfeeding benefits for mothers

Health providers advise new mothers to provide optimal health benefits to their babies by breastfeeding them for a year. Besides the provision of natural nourishment to infants, breastfeeding can also benefit their mothers in the following ways:

-Breastfeeding facilitates the return of the uterus to its size before pregnancy. While nursing in the first few weeks after birth, you may experience some mild contractions. This tightening sensation indicates that the uterus is shrinking. The oxytocin released during nursing helps the uterus to return to its previous size by triggering a contraction and reducing bleeding of the uterus.

-Aids you to shed pregnancy weight. The production of breast milk burns calories. Consequently, breastfeeding your baby can help you get rid of the extra calories gained during

pregnancy. Nursing mothers can slowly lose weight without dieting.

-*Reduces the risk of cancer.* Women who breastfeed have a lower risk of ovarian and breast cancers in their older age.

-*Natural birth control.* Though not reliable, frequent breastfeeding can delay ovulation and consequently menstruation. The prolactin released during breastfeeding hinders progesterone and estrogen from triggering ovulation. As a result, a nursing mother is likely to remain infertile until the level of prolactin drops and ovulation resumes.

Lactation amenorrhea provides a natural means of birth control. However, it is not as effective as other methods of birth control. Exclusive and frequent breastfeeding can help increase the production of prolactin and delay ovulation. Avoid the use of pacifiers and nurse your baby at night.

-*Risk of osteoporosis*. Breastfeeding may reduce the risk of osteoporosis in nursing mothers. The absorption of calcium occurs efficiently in pregnant and lactating women. The bones of these women are likely to be denser after nursing their babies than at the pre-pregnancy period.

Besides, breastfeeding allows a mother to spend time with her baby. Such awesome sessions encourage bonding between mother and child.

CHAPTER 2

GETTING STARTED

A woman's breasts produce small amounts of colostrum within 3-4 days after birth. This first milk is a yellowish fluid which is rich in antibodies and proteins. Besides providing passive immunity to newborns, the colostrum assists their digestive systems to function correctly. Frequent feedings of about 2hours intervals will stimulate the breasts to produce more milk.

During the 8-20 days of a baby's life, the breast milk changes in quantity, taste, and color. This transitional milk will give way to mature milk in the fourth week after birth.

The Right Moment To Start Breastfeeding

You can initiate breastfeeding within an hour after delivery. Babies tend to have strong desire to suckle within this period. Moreover, placing your newborn on your chest few minutes after delivery will help to calm the baby. The skin-to-skin contact will encourage the infant to breastfeed. When your baby is ready to suckle, guide him to make sure he latch onto the breast properly. (See "Guide To Making A Good Latch" on CHAPTER 4)

It is important to recognize a newborn's readiness to breastfeed. You can easily detect the feeding signals if you room-in with your baby after delivery. A newborn may give any of the following cues:

-He attempts to suck your finger if you place it at the corner of his mouth.

-The baby increases the movement of his eyes when they are open or closed.

-He chews his finger or any object that comes near his mouth.

-He moves his head and opens mouth to search for breast.

-The newborn makes sucking sounds.

Fidgeting is also an early hunger cue. However, mothers should pay attention to their babies to observe these signals. Always breastfeed when your baby wants to be fed. Babies may demand up to 15 feedings daily within the first week after birth. Frequent breastfeeding during this period can stimulate breast milk production. Do not reduce the frequency of the feedings.

Interval And Length Of Breastfeeding Session

Breast milk is a natural food which contains all the nutrients needed by newborns. Due to its unique properties, it is recommended as the only nourishment for babies until they are six months old. Mothers should continue breastfeeding after the exclusive nursing period. However, they can gradually introduce solid food to the infants.

Most newborns suckle 8 to 12 times daily from the third day after birth. They may continue with this number of feedings until they are six months old. The interval between the feedings varies since the babies are nursed on demand. It is ideal for mothers to wake their babies every two hours for breastfeeding in the first few weeks following delivery. You can allow the infant to sleep at night and nurse when he is hungry.

Babies do have long feedings with short intervals between the sessions when they desire. Most infants prefer to have this "cluster feedings" in the evenings. Though your baby may be fussy while nursing, but he is sucking enough milk to satisfy his hunger. Your baby may feel fuller after the closely spaced feedings. He can sleep for longer periods at night before demanding to be fed again.

The fat levels of the breast milk can make babies to vary their feedings. The amount of this nutrient during a feeding and from one nursing period to another can change. At the beginning of each breastfeeding session, the fat content of the breast milk is low.

However, it increases towards the end of the feeding as the milk becomes creamier. Babies are likely to sleep for more hours after cluster feeding due to intake of breast milk with higher fat levels.

During the early days of life, you should not wait for two hours to breastfeed your baby if he shows hunger cues. You can stop waking your baby for nursing when a pediatrician has confirmed that his growth rate is perfect. Then, breastfeed your baby when he demands for food.

It is not advisable to put a breastfeeding baby on schedule. Frequent nursing ensures healthy growth of a baby and increases milk production. Conversely, delaying the nursing session can result in poor weight gain in babies and low milk supply. The breasts will reduce their milk production if the time between consecutive feedings is much.

Babies can take 10 to 45 minutes to feed. A baby stops sucking on a breast for few minutes if he is satisfied. However, you can put him on the second breast if he wants to suck it. The baby gets creamier milk with more fat if he is allowed to suckle for longer periods on a breast. Consequently, you should not specify the time your baby spends on each breast.

Lactation Period

Due to its benefits and long-term impact on children, the WHO (World Health Organization) recommended exclusive breastfeeding for the first half year of life. It is ideal to continue with this natural nourishment for 12 months. Besides, a mother can breastfeed her child for more than a year if she desires to do so. After the six months of exclusive breastfeeding, it is advisable to introduce solid food to babies.

Some people believed that breastfeeding a baby for over a year provides no nutritional value to the infant. Contrary to this myth, research on breast milk showed an increased fat level in the milk produced by women lactating for over a year.

The energy content of breast milk produced during prolonged breastfeeding is sufficient for the requirements of toddlers. The levels of its components changes to satisfy the immunological and nutritional needs of a growing infant. Besides, continued lactation reduces the risks of allergies and sicknesses in babies.

Nursing an infant beyond a year also benefits mothers. It lowers the risks of ovarian, uterine and breast cancer. Breastfeeding a baby for more than six months is normal. The infant still obtains nutrients and more energy from the breast milk.

Also, it improves the health of the baby and mother. Since nursing can help mothers to burn up extra calories, prolonged lactation is a perfect means of losing weight after childbirth.

Breastfeeding positions

Despite being a natural activity, it may take time to master breastfeeding. However, practice will make it easier for you and your baby to master the skill. You can try various positions to determine the best for you and your baby. An ideal nursing position will be comfortable for both mother and baby. Also, it will allow the infant to latch properly on the breast.

However, you may need to change your preferred nursing position if it is no longer comfortable as your baby grows. Here are the common breastfeeding positions:

Cradle hold

Hold your baby with his stomach supported on your body. Position his head in the crook of your elbow while facing the breast on the side of the arm supporting his head. Align the infant's head with his entire body to avoid neck strain.

You may place a pillow across your laps for extra support.

A comfortable chair with armrests will be ideal for you to sit up and properly nurse your baby in this position. You can rest your elbow on the armrest or use a nursing pillow to make the position more comfortable. However, some moms may find it difficult to nurse their newborns in this position.

Cross-cradle position

This nursing position supports newborns to make a proper latch. You can also use it if your baby is finding it difficult to latch on the breast. It is the best option when both mother and baby are learning the act of breastfeeding.

Position your baby to have a tummy to tummy contact with you and opposite the nursing breast. Use the left arm to support your baby if you are breastfeeding from the right breast and vice versa.

Then, use your hand to support the base of his head. Hold your breast with the other hand, placing the thumb on top behind the areola and the fingers underneath. Without leaning forward, gently guide him to make a deep latch.

Football or clutch hold

It is an ideal breastfeeding position if you have delivered through a c-section as it keeps your abdomen free from the baby's weight. You can also use it for breastfeeding premature babies, twins, and newborns. Besides, women with large breasts can comfortably nurse their babies in this position.

Hold your baby just the way you hold a football or a clutch bag. Position your baby to face you while lying along your forearm while bending your elbow. Keep him at the same height as your waist and tuck his legs under your arm. With your index finger and thumb behind his ears, support his neck and head. Then use your free hand to hold your breast.

You can use a pillow for extra support and bring your baby to the level of your breast. However, you can place a pillow at either side of your body if you are nursing twins at the same time.

Side-lying position

This is an excellent nursing position for night feedings while in bed. It is also ideal if you are exhausted after childbirth or recovering from episiotomy or c-section. Mothers are likely to use this position if they co-sleep with their babies. The side-lying position allows you to rest while you feed your baby. A pillow under your head can keep you comfortable while nursing in this position.

While lying on your side, position your baby to lie down on his side alongside you and facing you. Place his head at the same level with your breast. With your free hand, hold your breast and take it to his mouth. When he correctly latches on the breast, use the hand to hold his neck and head while you support yourself on the other arm. You can also use a rolled-up towel or blanket to support your baby's back.

Some newborns may have difficulty nursing in a side-lying position. Besides, mothers who co-sleep with their babies should be careful while breastfeeding them in this position. It can increase the risk of suffocation in newborns. Remove all blankets and pillows near your before you feed your baby in this position. Better still; make sure you return him to his crib before you fall asleep especially if he is a newborn.

Laid-back or reclining position

This position helps nurse a baby with latching difficulties, a preemie or even twins. Besides, women recovering from childbirth or surgery can comfortably nurse their babies in the reclining position. It is ideal for the first breastfeeding after childbirth. This nursing position allows the newborn to find the nipple by reflex and latch on it. Consequently, it is also known as biological nurturing.

Make yourself comfortable in a reclining position as you lie back on a sofa or bed. You can use pillows to support your neck and head. Position your baby to have a belly to belly contact with you. Make sure that his head is at the same level with your breast. Allow the infant to find the nipple and latch on it. However, you may help the baby.

You can nurse an older baby, who can support his head in a sitting position. It is also good for babies who wriggle while nursing if feel restrained. Position your baby to sit upright with each of his legs on either side of your belly. However, you can support a younger infant with a slightly bent arm. Make sure that the baby's back and neck are aligned in a straight line and his nose is not covered while breastfeeding.

A single nursing position may not satisfy the needs of a baby and mother. Besides, changing breastfeeding positions can help you to empty your breasts. Always hold your baby near the breasts to prevent the infant from pulling on your nipple while breastfeeding. Position him with his body and head facing the same direction.

Make sure you sit up straight when you breastfeed your baby. Latching-on problems can result if you hunch over the baby while nursing. Your baby will get enough milk when he is properly positioned.

Tips for successful breastfeeding in any of the positions

You need to try out different nursing positions to find a suitable one for you and your baby.

Determine positions that are the best in different situations. You may need to change a nursing position to achieve a successful breastfeeding experience. Besides, you may need to change the preferred position as your baby become older.

A suitable breastfeeding position allows your baby to properly latch on the breast and nurse comfortably. It will also reduce pain, risk of injuries to the nipple and does not strain the muscles. The following tips will help you to breastfeed your baby in comfort.

Make yourself comfortable. Sit in a chair that has armrests. You may need pillows for extra support to your back and arms. Use a footstool to support your feet especially in the first few weeks after childbirth. You may use a coffee table or any other comfortable object to raise your feet.

Support your baby. Hold your baby in place with your hand or arm. You can bring his head to the level of your breast by placing a pillow or folded blanket under his back and head. You can also position your baby on top of a pillow placed on your lap. The extra support will make him more comfortable. Besides, it is an ideal option for mothers that had a c-section.

Support your breasts while breastfeeding. Use your hands to hold your breasts as they will be heavier when filled with milk. Make sure your fingers did not cover the areola and nipple so that the infant can make a good latch on the breast. Use a rolled-up blanket or towel to raise the nipple to the same height as your baby's mouth if your breasts are large.

Allow your baby to nurse on both breasts during each feeding session. Offer the second breast after the infant has drained the first one. Then, put him on the second breast first during the next feeding. Nursing your baby first on the full breast will help prevent mastitis and improve milk production.

Alternate breastfeeding positions during and between feedings. This practice can help prevent breast infection, plugged milk ducts,

and nipple soreness. The best positions will
enable you and your baby to have an enjoyable
breastfeeding   experience.

CHAPTER 3

BREASTFEEDING PROBLEMS

Breast milk is the best nourishment for newborns. Besides being a natural process, breastfeeding provides various health benefits to both baby and mother. Problems may arise during the lactation period. These difficulties can discourage a mother from nursing her baby. Consequently, some nursing mothers can't complete the recommended six months of exclusive breastfeeding.

Breastfeeding problems can interfere with an infant's ability to breastfeed or the production of breast milk. Dehydration and weight loss may result if the babies are not getting enough breast milk. Nursing mothers need support to enable them to breastfeed their newborns successfully.

Signs of Breastfeeding Problems

Early detection of any condition that will interfere with breastfeeding is crucial. You need to get help immediately you notice the problem.

Consult your baby's pediatrician for solutions if you observe any of the following signs.

-The baby is not gaining weight after two weeks or is under his birth weight. Such insufficient weight gain indicates that the baby is not sucking enough breast milk.

-Experiencing pain while breastfeeding. It may result from improper latching. Find out how to make a good latch in CHAPTER 4. Cracked nipples can also cause pain and discomfort. You can contact a lactation consultant or physician if the condition interferes with nursing.

-The infant shows hunger cues after most feedings. Your baby may not be sucking enough milk. Ensure that he latches onto the breast properly. Also, check the breastfeeding position as it may influence the quantity of milk your baby consumes. Consult the baby's pediatrician if the breast milk supply is low.

-The breasts are not filled with milk five days after delivery. Get your breasts examined if you didn't feel the milk let down. Weighing your baby will determine whether he is getting enough milk.

-Your baby may be experiencing ineffective suckling if the fullness of the breasts does not decrease after feedings.

-Your baby may not be getting enough milk if the breastfeeding sessions in the first few months are less than ten minutes. However, low milk production can cause infants to feed consistently for more than fifty minutes during feedings.

-Hard and painful breasts which can prevent breastfeeding. This condition may decrease the milk supply.

-Less than four stools and six wet diapers daily. The diaper changes during the early days of life can detect whether a baby is breastfeeding properly. Contact your pediatrician if the stool is still dark after one week or the urine is a deep yellow. At this period, the stool should be loose and yellow.

As a natural process, breastfeeding should be easy. With the right support, mothers can overcome difficulties and breastfeed their babies for longer periods. However, it is important for first-time mothers to learn how to breastfeed.

Preparing for Breastfeeding

During pregnancy, a woman's body prepares for breastfeeding. The breasts become tender and larger while the areolas get darker when a woman is pregnant. The tiny glands around the areolas produce oily substances that protect the breast. "Roughing up" your nipples can get rid of these protective materials and make them sore. Avoid rubbing the nipples with a towel.

You can give your breasts some gentle massage to enable you to get used to handling them.

Besides, it will be useful if you have to express your breast milk later manually. Gently stroke the entire breast in a circular pattern. Start from the upper part and move towards the nipple.

Check your breasts for inverted nipples. Your baby may find it difficult to correctly latch on to a nipple with an indentation at the middle. You can perform a pinch test to determine whether you possess inverted nipples. Use your forefinger and thumb to pinch your areolas. An inverted nipple will retract into the breast. The extent of the inversion varies from slight to severe. A physician or lactation consultant can confirm whether your nipples are flat or inverted.

A baby may experience difficulty in gripping a flat nipple. However, an expert can help solve the problem. Some women may have one protruding nipple and an inverted one. Many women who have inverted nipples can successfully breastfeed their babies.

They can use devices such as nipple enhancer, breast shells, and a breast pump to stimulate their nipples to pop out. Joining a breastfeeding support group will help women to learn how to use these tools properly.

Massaging an inverted nipple between the thumb and the forefinger can make it erect. You can stimulate the nipple to protrude before each feeding. Alternatively, you can squeeze the breast to pop out the nipple once your baby latches on to suck. If your baby finds it difficult to latch onto the breast, use a nipple shield. However, you have to consult a lactation specialist before using the device to ensure appropriate usage.

Use only water to keep your breasts clean. Soaps can make them dry. However, you can apply lubricants if your nipples are extremely dry. A lubricant can prevent your nipples from cracking. Breastfeeding can be painful if the nipples are cracked. Lotions are not necessary unless you have skin infections such as eczema. Ensure that you consult a physician for the right prescription for a breastfeeding mother.

First-time moms need support and advice from relatives and friends who have breastfed their children. Joining a breastfeeding support group will be helpful. It will encourage you to establish successful breastfeeding. Besides, you will learn from the experiences of other nursing mothers. You may meet women who had suffered from different breastfeeding problems such as engorged breasts, cracked nipples, and others. You can find a lactation forum online if there is none in your area.

Reading books can also help to prepare a woman mentally for breastfeeding. Books on pregnancy, childbirth, breastfeeding, nutrition, and parenting are helpful. Some lactation support groups lend these materials to encourage breastfeeding mothers.

You can consult a lactation specialist before the arrival of your baby if you have questions. The professional can also assist you in establishing successful breastfeeding after delivery. A lactation consultant can provide solutions to your nursing problems. Certified breastfeeding experts work privately or in hospitals.

CHAPTER 4

LATCHING PAIN

Breastfeeding mothers, especially the first-timers, may experience sore nipple at the initial stage of a nursing period. Such discomfort is normal when the baby first grips the nipples. If it persists during a breastfeeding session, it can make the process painful. Adjust the baby's position to help him latch properly. However, you can guide your baby to make a good latch.

Get your baby to release the nipples. You can insert your index finger in his mouth while tickling his chin to remove him from the breast. Then use the techniques described below to assist him in making a good latch. Ensure that his lips splay out and cover the areola after the latch. The baby's nose and chin should touch your breast. An improper latch can lead to nipple pain.

If breastfeeding still hurts when latching and positioning are appropriate, then, you may have dry nipples. Consult a physician or lactation specialists if the nipples have cracks to prevent infection. Use lanolin creams to lubricate them and avoid washing with soap. Putting on loose clothing can be helpful.

Women with flat or inverted nipples experience latching pain. Find out how to prepare such nipples for breastfeeding in the previous chapter. You can also contact a professional for help. Besides, the fullness of the breasts within the first couple of weeks after birth can flatten the nipples. Your newborn may find it difficult to latch during this period due to the firmness of your areolas.

In many women, nipple pain occurs as the baby grips a breast. It disappears a few minutes into the breastfeeding session. The letdown of milk as the infant sucks will ease the discomfort. Normally, latching pain will occur only for an instant if the milk flow to the nipples becomes quicker than at the beginning of the feeding. However, ensure that the baby latches properly.

Guide To Making A Good Latch

Though a natural act, breastfeeding is a learned behavior. Mothers, especially first-time moms need support to establish the right breastfeeding practices. Supportive ante-natal sessions can aid them to initiate breastfeeding and nurse their babies appropriately.

Proper latching of a baby onto the mother's breast is an important aspect of successful breastfeeding. Nursing could be painful if a baby did not make a good latch. An appropriate breastfeeding position is crucial for a newborn to make a proper latch. The following tips can help mothers to make sure their babies latch properly onto the breasts during nursing.

-Always hold your baby to have tummy-to-tummy contact with you.

-Do not lean on the infant. Such a position will strain your shoulder and neck.

-Make sure that the baby's nose is opposite the nipple.

-Hold the breast on both sides with one hand. Keep your fingers away from the nipple to ensure a perfect latch.

-Compress the breast if large by cupping it in a U-hold while keeping your fingers parallel to the baby's lip.

-Slightly tilt the baby's head back and touch his upper lip with the nipple. This action will make him open his mouth.

-The baby can properly latch onto the breast if his mouth is wide open with the tongue lowered. Rub the nipple over the upper lip again if the baby's mouth is not wide enough.

-Make sure that the baby's mouth covers the lower part of the areola. You can use a finger to pull down the lower lip if this area surrounding the nipple is not in the baby's mouth.

Your baby successfully suckles if he makes a good latch. Always hold your baby in the right position and make yourself comfortable during the feeding. You can use a breastfeeding pillow for support and maintain a proper feeding position. However, a mother can confirm a perfect latch with these signs:

-The baby's mouth covers the areola.

-The tongue is visible when you pull down the lower lip.

-The chin indents the lower part of the breast.

-Nipple soreness or discomfort diminishes while the baby breastfeeds.

-The baby does not make smacking noises.

-A swallowing rhythm as the infant draws out the milk.

Always position your baby well during nursing sessions (check CHAPTER 2 for breastfeeding positions). Help the infant to make a deep latch to enable him to drain the breast milk with ease and prevent nipple injuries.

CHAPTER 5

ENGORGED BREASTS

Women experience breast engorgement when milk overfills their breasts. This condition arises when a mother produces more milk than her baby consumes. In the first few weeks after delivery, tissue fluid and blood in the breasts can also lead to engorgement. Normally, the breasts feel hard, fuller, and larger in the first few days after birth. During this period, they produce more milk. Within two to three weeks following birth, the fullness reduces. The breasts become softer, but they can still produce abundant milk.

The fullness of the breasts becomes a problem when they are swollen and painful. The swelling of the throbbing breasts may reach your armpits. In some cases, the engorgement may result in low fever. Your baby may not grip the nipples properly if your breasts are engorged. In such a situation, the areola becomes hard.

You may experience pain in the nipples when your baby attempts to latch onto the breast. Prolonged engorgement can cause the body to produce less milk. Besides the low milk supply, engorgement can lead to severe health issues. You should contact a lactation consultant or physician if you have swollen, painful, and hard breasts.

Causes of engorgement

After giving birth, your milk produces colostrum which provides immune factors that will protect the newborn. This first milk is rich in nutrients needed by the baby. The quantity of the colostrum produced will be the right amount that will satisfy your newborn. Your breasts will start producing more milk 2 to 5 days after birth.

During this period, your breasts will become swollen, warm, firm, and heavy as more milk comes in. This condition known as engorgement is normal. It lasts for a few days and eases off as your body adjusts to the breastfeeding needs of your baby.

The exact period of engorgement depends on the individual. In some women, it may persist for a week or more. Despite breastfeeding regularly, your breast can still become swollen if your baby is sucking less milk than usual. The same condition will arise if the infant takes fewer feedings or stops breastfeeding.

Your breasts will be engorged if your baby doesn't empty the breasts while nursing. Many infants suck less milk when they start consuming solid foods than when they feed only on breast milk. Poor appetite due to ill health can also cause infants to breastfeed less.

Besides, you can have engorged breasts if you can't breastfeed your baby soon after birth. The swelling will gradually ease if you don't stimulate your breasts to produce more milk.

In some cases, the breasts become engorged if your baby misses a feeding or sleeps longer than usual. Nursing your newborn on a schedule or weaning him too quickly can also cause the breasts to swell. Pumping more milk

65

than your newborn requires can stimulate the breasts to produce more milk causing engorgement.

Obstructed milk ducts can cause engorged breasts. Such a situation may arise from breast augmentation. The implant may occupy much space in the breasts, leaving little room for the milk, and increased blood, and lymph. Wearing a tight bra or clothing can also block the ducts.

Despite how frequent and well your baby feeds, your breasts may still be engorged. Any condition that interferes with breastfeeding your baby on demand can lead to engorgement. However, gentle massage and regular breastfeeding can help empty the swollen breasts. You can also pump the milk to drain the swollen breasts.

Your baby may not be able to make a good latch if the breast is excessively full. The swelling makes the breast to become firm. Your baby will find it difficult to grasp the nipples. The infant will not be able to empty the breasts. This situation can increase the severity of the engorgement. Eventually, the breasts may become inflamed and painful.

You may also experience fever which may be a sign of infection. Consult a physician once your temperature rises if your breasts are engorged. Besides the fever that may arise from severe engorgement, the condition can also reduce milk production. The milk already in the swollen breasts induces the body to minimize its milk production. If not drained, this condition can lead to the weaning process.

Symptoms of breast engorgement

The following signs indicate that you have engorged breasts:

-Swollen, throbbing, and hard breasts.

-Firm areola and flattened nipples. Your baby may find it difficult to latch on the breast.

-The swelling extends to your armpits. The lymph nodes in that body part become tender and swollen.

-A slight increase in temperature (38 degrees Celsius).

In cases of severe engorgement, the breasts become badly swollen, firm, painful, and warm. The engorged breasts can cause the areola to be firm making it hard for your baby to grasp the nipples. Consequently, they may crack and become sore. The cracked nipples can worsen the condition. It may also lessen the frequency of breastfeeding. Prolonged breast engorgement prevents the baby from getting sufficient milk from the breasts. It can lead to mastitis (breast infection) and blocked milk ducts. You need to consult a doctor if the engorgement persists. Medical attention will prevent serious health issues.

Treatment of Breast Engorgement

You will enjoy breastfeeding your baby if you can ease the symptoms of engorgement. The following tips will help increase milk flow and relieve swollen breasts.

-Nurse your baby more frequently if your breasts are engorged. The intervals between the breastfeeding sessions should not be more than three hours. 8 to 12 feedings in a day can help empty the retained milk.

-Express the breast milk if your baby is sleeping when it is time for a feeding. Emptying the breast milk will ease the overly full milk ducts. You can easily express the milk manually with your hands in the shower.

-Hands express some milk to make it easy for your baby to latch on the breasts. Manual expression of breast milk softens the areola and makes it more flexible. If you pump an engorged breast, hand express it after pumping to enable your baby grip the areola easily. Keep the breast pump at its lowest setting before usage.

-Do not express your breast milk if your baby is breastfeeding well at intervals of two to three hours. Pumping the breasts in this situation can stimulate them to produce more milk. Prolonged breast engorgement and overproduction of milk can result from excessive pumping. However, you can hand express a little to soften the breasts.

-A gentle massaging of the breasts while your baby breastfeeds will increase the milk flow. Lightly rub each breast as your baby sucks on it. This action not only facilitates emptying of the breasts but it also relieves pain and the firmness of the engorged breasts.

-A warm shower just before a breastfeeding session can also increase the milk flow. Applying a warm compress on the breasts for three minutes is also helpful. Make sure that you don't prolong the duration of use to prevent further swelling. However, avoid heat application in cases of severe engorgement. Don't use warm compresses if the milk isn't flowing out.

-You can apply cold packs to your swollen breasts to ease the swelling and throbbing. After nursing your baby, place a plastic bag containing crushed ice on each breast for ten minutes. You can also use a bag of frozen vegetables or frozen wet towel. Ideally, spread a thin cloth on your breast before placing the cold compress to avoid damaging your skin. Placing chilled cabbage leaves under a tight shirt or inside your bra can minimize inflammation.

-Relaxation techniques can also relieve engorgement. Fluids in the swollen breasts will drain away if you rest while lying flat on your back.

-A supportive and well-fitted nursing bra can make you feel better. However, make sure that the bra has no underwire to avoid clogged ducts.

-Acetaminophen or ibuprofen can reduce the swelling and pain. Though these medications are safe to take while breastfeeding, you have to contact your physician for directions.

-Contact a doctor if your temperature increases to 101 degrees Fahrenheit or above. Fever is an indication of a breast infection.

Prevention of breast engorgement

Some women experience full breasts just for a few days after birth. It is normal for the breasts to become engorged during this period due to the increase in breast milk production. Conversely, this condition persists in some women leading to swollen, hard, and painful breasts. The ideas below will help you to avoid prolonged breast engorgement.

-Put your newborn to the breast as soon as possible after birth. Health professionals recommend initiating breastfeeding within a baby's first two hours of life. It will give your baby time to learn how to feed on the breasts before they become overfilled with breast milk (Find out how to start breastfeeding in CHAPTER 2 of this book)

-Avoid breastfeeding your baby on a schedule. It is ideal to breastfeed a newborn 8 to 12 times in the first few weeks after birth. Though your baby may have fewer feedings in the first 24 hours after delivery, you have to nurse him frequently. Skin to skin contact with your baby can stimulate him to breastfeed.

-Feed your baby on demand. Try to recognize his hunger cues as discussed in CHAPTER 2. You can wake your baby for feeding if three hours have elapsed after the last session.

-Make sure your baby latches on the breast well. A proper latch and position will enable him to empty the breasts and prevent retention of produced breast milk.

-Allow your baby to finish sucking one breast before you put him on the other. Let him nurse on the second breast when you no longer hear the swallowing sounds, or he stops sucking the first one. However, if he did not nurse long on the second breast, put him on it first during the next feeding.

-Pump or hand express your milk to empty your breasts if your baby doesn't feed well or skips a feeding.

-Don't supplement breastfeeding with formula. Feed your baby expressed breast st milk if your lactation consultant or physician recommends supplementing with a bottle.

-Don't introduce a pacifier or bottle in the first month after birth. However, you can do so if your doctor recommends it for medical reasons. Your baby may find it difficult to suck the breasts if he gets used to feeding on a bottle. Such a situation affects the quantity of milk he sucks during nursing (See "nipple preference").

-Wean your baby gradually to avoid retaining much milk in your breasts.

Breast engorgement makes it hard for your baby to grip the areola. Consequently, he may not get enough milk during the feedings. This condition eases up within 2 to 5 days in most women. If it persists, the retained milk will lead to swollen, hard, and painful breasts. The resulting sore and cracked nipples interfere with breastfeeding. Emptying the engorged breasts is crucial to avoid breast infection. Also, try to reduce the swelling and pain.

Consult your physician if the engorgement is severe. If left untreated, low milk supply, plugged milk ducts, breast abscess, and mastitis may result.

CHAPTER 6

PLUGGED DUCTS

A milk duct can become blocked, clogged, or plugged if it doesn't drain properly. This problem arises when a breast becomes overfull with milk for some time. The milk ducts are small tube-like structures through which the milk flows to the nipple. They form a branching network that converges at the nipple. The squeezing action of the muscles on these ducts facilitates the milk flow during breastfeeding.

When your breast produces more milk than the quantity emptied during nursing, the ducts will retain the excess. The accumulation of milk in the breast can lead to the swelling of the tissues surrounding the ducts. The inflamed muscles press on these tubes, hindering the milk flow. Eventually, the backup of breast milk in the ducts result in a blockage.

Besides the obstruction of the milk ducts, the blockage may also occur in the nipple pore. This breastfeeding problem affects only one breast at a time. However, many nursing mothers experience this type of inflammation due to the extended periods between breastfeeding sessions. Also, pressure from the baby carrier or tight bra can obstruct the free flow of breast milk through the ducts. The pain resulting from a clogged milk duct can spread throughout the affected breast.

This painful condition can lead to reduced milk flow from the affected breast. It can also result in the presence of fat grains in breast milk. The breast milk accumulated due to the blockage of the ducts thickens.

Causes of a clogged duct

Plugged milk duct results if your breasts do not drain completely during feedings. The poor drainage of breast milk can lead to the development of clogs. This condition can hinder the normal flow of breast milk. Most cases of clogged duct occur in the first few weeks after birth. During this period, both the mother and newborn are getting used to the act of breastfeeding. Eventually, the quantity of breast milk produced will depend on your baby's needs. The blockage of the milk ducts can also result from the following situations.

-A sudden change in your baby's breastfeeding schedule. Irregular feedings can lead to the back up of milk. Your baby may sleep through a feeding, extending the usual interval between

the sessions. Besides, you may not be able to feed your baby frequently if you are sick. Pump your breast milk if your baby misses a feeding especially at night. Emptying the breasts will help prevent clogged ducts.

-*Incomplete draining of the breast.* An improper latch can hinder your baby from nursing properly. If the infant doesn't empty the breasts after feedings, the accumulated milk can form a clog. Pump your breasts to drain them if the need arises.

-*Abrupt weaning.* Gradually stop breastfeeding your baby to allow your body to adjust to the reduced feedings. Rapid weaning can lead to the accumulation of breast milk and consequently a clog.

-*Compression of the milk ducts.* Baby carriers, wearing tight clothing or bra can exert pressure continuously on the breasts obstructing the milk flow. Such a situation can lead to the formation of a clog. Sleeping on your stomach can also have the same effect on the ducts.

-*Fatigue.* Stress can lead to exhaustion. If you are tired, your body will find it difficult to facilitate milk flow. Such a situation can result in poor drainage of breast milk and the development of a clog. Also, stress lowers the production of the hormone, oxytocin. This chemical compound stimulates the release of milk from a woman's breasts.

-*A bleb or blocked nipple pore.* A tiny whitish-yellow obstruction at a duct's opening on the nipple can hinder the breast milk from flowing out. Such a spot might result from the accumulation of the milk's fatty residue. It may also be an overgrowth of your skin cells. This area hurts when your baby sucks the affected breast.

-*Breast biopsy.* The part of the breast operated upon can hinder milk flow. Consequently, blockage of the milk ducts may occur due to the back up of milk.

-Feeding position. Your breast milk may not empty if you always keep your baby in the same position while nursing. The milk left in the ducts after the feedings can cause a blockage.

Consult your doctor immediately you notice a clogged nipple. It may degenerate to mastitis if left untreated.

Symptoms of clogged ducts

A blocked duct can occur as a painful lump in the affected breast. It may also exist as a tender and swollen patch on the breast. The sore swelling may be reddish. When a lump results from a plugged duct, its size can vary from the size of a dime to that of a peach.

The following signs indicate that you might have a plugged duct.

-A tender spot or hard lump in your breast.

-Soreness and redness of the affected part.

-Inflammation or hot sensation that may ease a little after a breastfeeding session.

-Fever can occur if the blocked duct becomes infected. Mastitis may set in if the condition is left untreated. You should consult a physician immediately you experience high temperatures.

The position of the blockage may shift. However, the feeling of fullness may persist after nursing due to the accumulated milk behind the obstruction. Breastfeeding your baby on the affected breast can help reduce the throbbing and swelling caused by the plugged duct.

Treatment of a clogged duct

The inflammation and pain experienced in the affected breast will reduce if you unclog the milk duct. Though the swelling will ease the area may remain tender and reddish for some days. Here are tips that can aid you to free your milk ducts of blockages.

Frequent breastfeeding

Nursing your baby on the affected breast may be painful, but it is necessary to empty it. Breastfeeding more frequently than the regular feedings can help drain the breast. Always nurse your baby first on the breast with blocked ducts. It may help dislodge the clog as babies tend to suck the strongest at the start of a feeding.

Vary the nursing position to improve the drainage. However, ensure that your baby makes a good latch. You could pump or express the milk if your baby did not empty the affected breast. Pumping the milk will fully drain the breast and prevent further clogging.

Switch breastfeeding positions

Changing your baby's position during feedings can improve breast milk drainage. If you use a clutch hold, change to cross-over or cradle position. Good positioning can improve suction and help free a plugged duct. Make sure your baby points his chin in the direction of the sore spot before he latches on the breast.

Moist heat application

Moist heat is effective in loosening a clog in the milk duct. Taking several hot showers each day or applying wet and warm compresses to the sore area can ease discomfort, swelling, and pain. Apply moist heat to the affected breast before nursing your baby.

Massage

Gentle and frequent massages of the sore spot can be helpful. Use your thumb to rub the area. Start from behind the clog and move towards the nipple. Careful massaging from the edge of the blockage can help dislodge it and improve the milk flow.

Rest and feed well

Relax and get some sleep. It may be difficult if you have other children besides your newborn. However, a relative can help you take care of your kids a few hours daily while you take a nap. Intake of more fluids will keep you hydrated. Besides, the consumption of nutritious foods can improve your immune system.

Medications

You may take ibuprofen to ease the pain and swelling. However, you should consult a lactation consultant or your physician to avoid breast milk interaction with the drug.

Prevention of clogged ducts

Blocked milk ducts are painful and can interrupt breastfeeding. However, some measures can help check this nursing problem.

-Breastfeed your baby regularly to avoid engorgement. You can express your milk manually or use a pump if your baby doesn't empty your breasts after feeding. Avoid long

intervals between nursing sessions. Continuous breastfeeding is the best way to unclog blocked ducts.

-Switching your nursing position can improve milk flow. The sucking action of your baby can evenly drain milk from your breasts if you change his pose during feedings.

-Protect your breasts from pressure. Any object that presses on your breasts for an extended period can lead to the formation of a clog. Don't wear tight clothing. Avoid bras with underwire. They can compress milk ducts. You can wear a bigger sized bra for the time being. You may decide to go braless while at home. Also, avoid sleeping on your stomach.

-Massaging and use of moist heat after each nursing session can help prevent the formation of plugs in the milk ducts. It can also ease pains resulting from breastfeeding.

-Use warm water to gently wash off any dried milk blocking the openings in your nipples.

-Boost your immune system. Consumption of nutritious foods can improve your immunity. It is necessary to increase your Vitamin C and fluid intake while breastfeeding your baby. This healthy habit will also energize your muscles.

Breast and nipple pains can interfere with your decision to provide your newborn with natural nourishment. You can still nurse your baby if you have clogged ducts. However, the infant may fuss during feedings due to the reduced milk flow.

Consult a physician or lactation consultant if clogged ducts persist. Remember to call for help, once your temperature rises. Fever can be an indication of infection.

CHAPTER 7

SORE NIPPLES

Many women have sore nipples in the early days of breastfeeding after birth. Some nursing mothers may think that this condition is normal while nursing. However, it is not so. You may experience some tenderness or pain for a few seconds when your baby starts to nurse in the first week after birth. This discomfort is not supposed to last throughout the feedings.

Usually, sore nipples can make breastfeeding uncomfortable. The sucking action of your baby may increase the discomfort. This situation will improve when your milk comes in within few days after birth. Besides, proper positioning of your baby and a good latch during feedings can prevent the nipple pain.

Persistent nipple soreness after you have established breastfeeding is not normal. Consult a lactation counselor if the soreness persists through feedings. Breastfeeding may become unbearable if the nipples begin to crack and bleed.

Causes of sore nipples

Several factors can lead to nipple soreness. The early manifestation of this nursing condition commonly results from a shallow latch and position. Ineffective sucking can also result in discomfort during breastfeeding. However, the following culprits can cause sore nipple in breastfeeding mothers.

-*Improper latch*: Nipple soreness is common in the early days of breastfeeding due to the inability of babies to make a good latch. You will experience pain if your baby sucks on the nipple instead of the breast.

Such a shallow latch can lead to nipple damage as your baby can't get enough of the breast into his mouth during breastfeeding. The soreness is intense when your baby first latches on the breast. However, the discomfort may continue throughout the feeding if the damage to the nipple is severe.

The suction will be more effective during nursing if the nipple is touching the back of your baby's tongue. Guide your baby to make a deeper and better latch. A lactation consultant can instruct you on how to position your baby to grip the breast and suck effectively.

-*Tongue-tie*: Your baby can't make a good latch if the frenulum extends to the front of his tongue or is short. The frenulum is the skin connecting the tongue to the bottom of the mouth. An experienced health professional can carry out a minor procedure to snip this skin. You can consult a lactation counselor, physician or midwife to check whether your baby is tongue-tied if you experience nipple discomfort while nursing.

-*Thrush*: This yeast infection not only causes pain but also damages the affected nipples. You may contact thrush if your baby has the fungal infection in his mouth. The condition manifests as white patches on the gum, tongue, and other inner surfaces of an infant's mouth. Breastfeeding moms suffering from thrush experience sharp pains in their nipples or breasts during and after nursing. Consult a physician for medical treatment if you and your baby have a thrush infection.

-*Nipple blister*: Swelling on the nipple filled with clear, bloody, and yellowish liquid, can cause intense pain during nursing. Suction from a shallow latch or use of breast pumps at high settings often leads to the formation of blisters on nipples. Friction from ill-fitting breast shields can also cause the same problem.

Application of medications, creams or ointments on nipples may cause reactions leading to contact dermatitis. This condition can result in the formation of blisters. Discontinue the use of any topical formulation if you have a nipple blister. However, you can consult a dermatologist to determine the cause of the blister.

Stop breastfeeding your baby once a blister develops on your nipple if you have previously suffered from herpes. The swelling may be a herpes lesion. Your baby can contract the virus if you nurse him on a breast with herpes affected nipple or areola. Breastfeed from the healthy breast only until the sore on the affected breast heals.

Emptying the breast with herpes lesion is necessary to avoid engorgement. You can pump and discard the milk since it is not safe for your baby's consumption. Consult your physician or lactation counselor once you have a nipple blister.

-*Milk bleb*: Breast milk can get trapped and block a duct if a layer of skin grows over the duct opening. This outgrowth (bleb) may appear as a yellowish or whitish dot on the nipple. A breastfeeding mother can feel pain on and behind a milk bleb. Your physician can peel the skin from the duct opening to treat the bleb. However, it may take weeks to heal if left on its own.

-*Breast pump trauma*: Nipple pain may also result from the use of a breast pump with ill-fitting breast shields or flanges. Don't express your milk with a breast pump that has shields that are too small for your nipples.

Also, you will experience nipple discomfort if the suction level of the pump is too high. Learn how to use a breast pump correctly. Always use a breast pump with well-fitting breast shields. You can contact a lactation consultant for assistance.

-*Vasospasm*: Fungal infection or poor latching can irritate the blood vessels in the nipple. The trauma causes the nipple to hurt and look pale after nursing. A spasm of the nipple's blood vessels can cause a burning sensation a few minutes after a feeding. The pain may last for some minutes before the nipple returns to its usual color. The process repeats itself as a throbbing sensation sets in which causes the nipple to become pale again.

The nipple turns white due to the spasm in the blood vessels and regains its normal color when the vessels relax. This condition called Raynaud's syndrome or vasospasm can affect both nipples at the same time. Exposure to cold can trigger a spasm in the blood vessels of a nipple.

You need to consult a physician for treatment if you are experiencing vasospasm. However, your lactation consultant can advise you on how to manage to breastfeed if you are suffering from this condition.

Caring for Nipple Soreness

The following tips can help soothe the tender nipple skin and facilitate the healing process.

-Keep your nipples dry. Make sure the skin of the affected nipple is free from moisture when you aren't nursing. You can use a soft and clean cotton cloth to pat it dry after each feeding. Besides, air-drying will be an ideal option if patting the nipple hurts. You can go braless or leave your shirt open and free your nipples from the bra flaps. Sleep on a towel at night if you are without a bra to absorb leaking milk.

Breastfeeding pads can trap moisture against the nipple. They can stick on the sore nipples causing more damage. If you need to use them, use those without plastic liners to avoid keeping the nipple skin moist. After each feeding, use dry and fresh breast pads.

Avoid using a hairdryer or any other quick-drying method to dry your nipple. Even on a low setting, the heat from this device can dry and crack the skin of more delicate nipples.

-*Exposure to air*. Unless you have vasospasm, exposing your nipples to air will aid healing. However, exposure of affected nipples to sunshine shouldn't exceed three minutes daily to avoid sunburn.

-Use of expressed milk. Gently massage a few drops of your breast milk into the tender skin of your nipples after each feeding. Besides stimulating circulation, it soothes the sore nipples and supports healing. The colostrum, which contains antibodies, is perfect nipple cream.

-The application of purified lanolin ointment. After feedings, spread a small amount of modified lanolin over your nipples to soothe them. Make sure that nipples are dry before applying it. The ointment promotes healing, prevents the formation of scab and helps the skin of the nipples and areola to retain their natural moisture. Lanolin also prevents

cracking of the nipples. Once you applied the ointment, you don't need to air dry the nipples.

Don't use creams and oils that you will need to wash off before nursing. Those formulations are not safe for your baby.

-Avoid washing your nipples regularly. Daily bathing is enough to keep it clean. Soaps remove natural oils secreted from glands on the areola. These oils lubricate and cleanse the area around your nipple, preventing dryness and cracking.

-Avoid friction on your nipples. Don't wear tight-fitting clothes or bra. They can compress your nipples. Instead, wear blouses or T-shirts

made from soft materials. You can also go braless.

-*Use of breast shells*. These plastics can prevent your sore nipples from rubbing on the bra fabric. Use dome-shaped shells with large holes to provide enough space for your nipples and prevent friction. You can wear breast pads over the shells if your breast milk leaks. A lactation specialist can help you choose breast shells that best suit your nipples.

Keep breastfeeding your baby while trying the remedies that will improve the discomfort. Nurse him first on the breast with the least soreness and then switch to the other one. Express your milk if the pain is unbearable and you can breastfeed. It is ideal to use a cup to feed your baby the expressed milk rather than using a rubber nipple.

The use of nipple shields may seem to be a nice option. However, suction through this device can cause the nipple to crack. They may also interfere with your baby's sucking action. These artificial nipples can make it harder for him to empty your breasts, effectively. Consequently, your breast supply will reduce.

Manage to breastfeed with sore nipples

Continue nursing your baby to maintain your breast milk supply. Allow him to first suck on the breast that hurts less and then switch to the other side. You can also seek the help of a lactation consultant or physician.

However, breastfeeding will be more comfortable when your baby's latch-on and sucking techniques improve. The following tips will make nursing less painful while the sore nipples heal.

-Assist your baby to make a deeper latch. Proper positioning will help your baby to grasp the nipples efficiently. Bring him close to your breast on his side and at the same level with your nipple. Make sure his mouth is wide-open

113

before he latches on the breast. Assist your baby to take in both the nipple and areola into his mouth.

Support the breast underneath with your fingers and on top with your thumb to keep its weight from your baby. Sandwiching your breast behind the areola will also help your baby to take more of the breast into his mouth. Flatten the breast tissues with your fingers and thumb while pushing back to make the areola narrower and longer. This adjustment will make your baby take in more of the areola inside his mouth.

-Prevent your baby from tight-mouthing your breasts. Push down your baby's chin with the

114

index finger of the hand you are using to support the breast. The pressure will keep his mouth wide open as he latches on the breast. It will also prevent him from gripping the sore nipple tightly throughout the feeding. Despite the nipple soreness, the mild pressure on your baby's chin will help you to nurse him more comfortably.

-Check your baby's sucking technique. Your baby's lips should turn out while sucking. Gently pull out his lower lip if he didn't turn it out when he latched on the breast. Soreness will develop underneath the nipples if he sucks in his lower lip.

-Make sure your baby's tongue is positioned properly while sucking. It should cup under the nipple to promote effective suction. Your nipples can become sore from breastfeeding if his tongue is backward and up in his mouth while sucking. Take him off the breast and position his tongue correctly.

During latch on, gently press your baby's chin down with the index finger of the hand you are using to support your breast. It will help to bring the tongue forward and down. Taking the breast with a wide-open mouth helps the tongue to protrude forward.

Your baby may be tongue-tied if his tongue is downward but can't cup under the breast.

Besides, it can stick out over the lower gum when his mouth is wide open. You can consult a physician about correcting the condition.

-Switch breastfeeding positions between feedings. It will help to reduce the discomfort resulting from the sore nipples during nursing. Many breastfeeding mothers find it easy to use the cross-cradle hold during the early days of breastfeeding. You can also use the clutch hold, cradle hold, or the side-lying position.

-Nurse on the least sore breast first. Then switch to the tender breast to empty its milk and maintain the supply. It is better to feed him on the breast that hurts more when his sucking has become less vigorous. Besides you can

117

nurse your baby more frequently, say every two to three hours.

You will experience less discomfort from the sore nipples if the feedings are shorter and more frequent. Regular breastfeeding will also prevent engorgement and maintain your breast milk supply.

-*Break the suction when the feeding is over.* It hurts if you take your baby off the breast when he is still sucking. It can lead to nipple soreness. To disrupt the suction, gently press down the breast near the baby's mouth. Your action will make him release the nipple in his mouth. Alternatively, you can insert your little finger into the corner of his mouth. However, make sure that your finger is clean.

Avoid the use of artificial nipples and pacifiers during the early days of breastfeeding. Your baby is learning to breastfeed and may develop nipple confusion. He may have problems latching and sucking on the breast if he gets used to suction techniques of feeding bottles.

Prevention of sore nipples

-Wear well-fitting and supportive bra.

-Help your baby to make a better and deeper latch.

-Change your baby's nursing position between feedings. Consult a lactation specialist for assistance if you can't hold your baby comfortably while breastfeeding.

Usually, your breasts may become sore from breastfeeding in the first few days or weeks postpartum. However, other causes such as fungal infection can prolong the soreness or cause it after weeks or months of painless breastfeeding. Contact a physician or lactation consultant to diagnose the cause of your nipple soreness and determine an effective treatment plan.

CHAPTER 8

CRACKED NIPPLES

Breastfeeding shouldn't be painful. Mothers suppose to nurse their babies comfortably and with pleasure. However, you may experience discomfort in the early weeks of breastfeeding. The nipple pain disappears when your baby learns to make a good latch and suck effectively. Sometimes, the soreness may worsen leading to nipple damage. The poor attachment of your baby to the breast can cause cracks to develop on the nipples.

These fissures may be visible on the skin of the nipple or between the areola and the nipple. A cracked nipple is painful and may bleed when you breastfeed your baby. The distress and pain resulting from this condition can cause new moms to quit breastfeeding. However, an adjustment of your baby's breastfeeding position and latching can help prevent further damage to the nipples.

Consult a lactation consultant without delay if you notice cracks on your nipples or that they bleed during nursing. The specialist can identify the cause of the problem and help to rectify it. Then, you will nurse your baby without pain.

You may experience a condition called "rusty pipe syndrome" that occurs in the early days of breastfeeding. A painless discharge of colored milk, which is a mixture of colostrums and a small amount of blood is its common sign. The breast milk becomes rust-colored, brown, pink or orange due to the presence of blood.

This colored milk isn't dangerous to the baby. You may not notice the change in color unless your newborn spits the milk or you are pumping it. A little blood may also occur in your baby's bowel due to the consumption of the colored milk.

However, the condition is temporary and disappears in just a few days without treatment. The "rusty pipe syndrome" is different from bleeding resulting from cracked nipples.

Causes of cracked nipples

Just like nipple soreness, most cases of cracked nipples result from inappropriate positioning and latching. However, there are other causes of this breastfeeding problem.

-Using a breast pump the wrong way. Setting the suction at high levels or using ill-fitting breast shields (flanges) can damage the nipple tissues causing cracks on the nipples. A flange is too small if your nipple can't move freely in it. Always use the right size of breast shields. Cracks or bleeding can also result from excessive suction from a breast pump. Consult your lactation consultant to guide you on how to use the breast pump correctly.

-Severe dry skin or eczema can lead to cracked nipples. Eczema occurs as red or scaly patches on the skin. It may be painful or itchy. Also, eczema-like condition (contact dermatitis) may result from the application of creams or ointments on the nipple. Consult a

dermatologist if you suspect that you have eczema.

-*Thrush.* It is a fungal infection that affects the mouth. You could contract thrush from your baby's mouth or infect him if you got it on your breast first. You will experience pains in your breast during and after nursing if you have this yeast infection. Besides, the affected nipples will become red, shiny and itchy.

-*Your baby can't latch properly if he is tongue-tied.* This condition can lead to ineffective suction and nipple damage. Your lactation consultant should examine your baby to confirm or rule out the possibility of a tongue-tie if you have cracked nipples.

Caring for cracked nipples

It is necessary to find out the cause of this nursing problem to prevent further damage to the nipple. The tips for treating nipple soreness are also effective if your nipples have cracks or bleed (Caring for sore nipples, Chapter 7). However, you may stop breastfeeding your baby on the breast that hurts more for a day if the pain is unbearable. Resting the nipple will help it to heal faster.

During this period, express your milk to keep up its supply and prevent engorgement. Then feed your baby the expressed milk. Gradually, resume nursing on the healing nipples. Frequent and short feedings will put less pressure on the breast. Breastfeeding every two to three hours is ideal. Regular feedings will prevent your baby from sucking aggressively.

Also, his suction will exert less pressure on the breast if you pump or hand express before letdown. Nurse your baby on the less sore breast and switch to the other side when he is less hungry. However, make sure that you position your baby properly to make a good latch. Breastfeeding should be painless if your baby takes a mouthful of both the areola and nipple.

You can lessen the pain if you numb the damaged nipple by applying a cold pack briefly to it before breastfeeding. Taking a pain reliever about 30 minutes before breastfeeding can reduce the swelling and pain. You need to consult a doctor for medications that are compatible with breastfeeding such as Acetaminophen and Ibuprofen. Make sure you follow the instructions concerning the dosage to avoid taking an overdose.

You can soothe your injured nipples by applying warm and moist compresses such as a wet washcloth or tea bags. Avoid using lotions, perfumes or alcohol, on your nipples. You can use clean water to rinse your breast after each feeding to minimize the risk of infection on the cracked nipple. However, you can clean the sore with a non-perfumed soap once a day and rinse adequately with water.

Your physician will prescribe an antibacterial ointment if you have an open wound. Consult your doctor as soon as possible if the sore isn't healing as expected. You will also need prescriptions for medications if the cracked nipple resulted from a medical condition.

Preventing cracked nipples

Breastfeeding can be pain-free. Always check your baby's attachment to avoid injuring your nipples. Make sure that he has a mouthful of both the nipple and areola with his chin pressing into the breast. A deeper latch will prevent friction on the nipples from the suction. It will also enable your baby to drain the calorie-rich hindmilk which supports weight gain.

Use a well-fitting nursing bra to avoid compressing your nipples. Don't wear tight-fitting clothes that can put pressure on your breast. If you must pump your milk, use a medical-grade breast pump. Your lactation counselor can help you to make the right choice. Also, learn how to use it correctly.

Breastfeeding while you have cracked nipples

The condition can't prevent you from nursing your baby. Apply the remedies for cracked nipples and continue nursing your baby while the sore heals. However, you may rest the nipples for 24 hours or so if breastfeeding is unbearable. Pump your milk and feed your baby with a flexible cup, medicine dropper or spoon.

Don't use a bottle to feed him the expressed milk. It will make his attachment to the breast poorer when he resumes nursing. He will latch on the breast, in the same manner; he takes the artificial nipples on the bottle. Besides interfering with your baby's latching technique, nipple confusion can prevent him from getting enough milk from the breasts.

Open wounds can easily get infected. Consult a physician right away if the cracks show signs of infection such as pus or inflammation, or if you develop a fever.

CHAPTER 9

MASTITIS

Some breastfeeding moms who experienced plugged ducts complained of fever when the condition persists. If you have a clogged milk duct that doesn't improve after 48 hours, visit a physician or lactation consultant right away.

134

Mastitis or breast infection can develop if you have a plugged duct. The lump on the breast will increase in redness or size. Also, you will experience severe pain and heat on the affected breast.

Mastitis commonly develops when bacteria grow within breast milk trapped in the ducts. Usually, it affects only one breast at a time, but it can develop in both. This condition is common during the first few weeks after birth. However, it can occur at any time during the lactation period or even after weaning your baby. An untreated breast infection can lead to a breast abscess, which is a collection of pus.

Causes of mastitis

Mastitis is an inflammation of the breast which commonly results from the blockage of milk ducts and engorgement. Milk stasis (milk left in the ducts after a feeding) is also a primary cause of breast infection. This condition can result from the obstruction of milk flow. Pump your breast after nursing your baby if he doesn't empty it.

Infection can also cause mastitis. Bleeding or cracked nipples can act as points of entry for harmful organisms. Sores on the nipple can increase the risk of infection. Besides, anemia, allergy, fatigue weakened immunity and stress can also lead to mastitis.

Symptoms of mastitis

Mastitis makes nursing mothers feel ill. The symptoms can manifest gradually or suddenly. They can be similar to a plug but with severe inflammation, heat, and pain. Signs of mastitis include the following:

-Pain while breastfeeding

-Swollen breast

-Skin redness on the affected breast

-Fever (101ºF or above)

-Chills

-Fatigue

Mastitis may lead to low milk supply in the swollen breast but it will not you're your baby.

Consult your doctor immediately you start experiencing these signs or flu-like symptoms.

Treatment of mastitis

Your lactation consultant or physician may recommend the following home treatments when the symptoms develop.

-Frequent breastfeeding. Nurse your baby frequently. Every two to three hours will be ideal if he is eager to suck. Though it will be painful, emptying the affected breast is crucial in the treatment of mastitis. Regular

breastfeeding will prevent blockage of milk ducts and maintain your milk supply.

During each feeding, nurse your baby first on the affected breast. Allow him to drain it completely if possible. Express or pump some milk if the breast is firm. Remove enough milk to soften the breast and enable your baby to grip the nipple easily and properly. Correct positioning will also help him to make a good latch.

Switching your breastfeeding positions during each feeding will help to empty the swollen breast. Pumping or manual expression of your milk will be helpful if your baby isn't draining it completely after nursing. Besides, you can pump your milk and bottle feed your baby with it, if the pain is unbearable during nursing.

You can express your milk but nursing your baby can empty your breast better than a suction device. Despite the pain, you can try and breastfeed your baby regularly. However, you can control the pain with medications and compresses.

-*Rest*. Stay in bed and relax. Get someone to assist with the household chores. Focusing on your recovery will be helpful. Stress and fatigue can also make you vulnerable to recurrent mastitis after recovery.

-*Warm and moist heat*. Before each feeding, take a hot shower or place a warm compress on the swollen breast. The heat will facilitate your milk flow and make breastfeeding less painful.

-*Cold compresses.* Apply a cold pack on the affected breast between the nursing sessions to ease swelling and pain. Always wrap the cold compress in a towel or clean cloth before use to avoid skin damage.

-*Avoid pressure on your breasts.* Tight clothing or bra can increase the swelling. You can go braless or wear loose bras. Avoid resting your baby on your chest or sleeping on your stomach.

-*Gentle massage.* Tenderly rub the swollen area of the affected breast. Massage towards the nipple and then move back to your armpit.

-*Medications*: Consult your physician to prescribe anti-inflammatory medicine. Over the counter medications like ibuprofen can provide relief from fever and pain. You need to start antibiotic treatment immediately if both breasts are swollen and your baby is less than two weeks old.

Medications are also vital for infectious mastitis. The following factors will suggest when to begin immediate treatment with antibiotics.

-A sudden increase in temperature.

-Severe symptoms of mastitis.

-Presence of a red streaking near a plug.

-Presence of pus or blood in breast milk.

-A cracked nipple that seems infected.

Typical antibiotics for treatment of mastitis include ciprofloxacin, cloxacillin, erythromycin, and nafcillin. These medications will not affect your breastfeeding baby. However, you have to consult a doctor for professional advice and prescriptions.

Make sure you are in contact with your lactation consultant or doctor who can monitor your recovery. Your physician may prescribe an antibiotic if there are signs of infection or the pain increases. You should complete the dosage even when the symptoms improve a couple of days after taking the medications. The

143

condition may reoccur if you haven't fully recovered and didn't take the prescribed amount of antibiotics.

Your doctor may recommend a different antibiotic if there is no improvement. However, avoid taking medications without a physician's prescription to avoid incompatibility with breastfeeding.

All cases of mastitis do not require antibiotics. Frequent emptying of the affected breast can facilitate milk flow and resolve non-infectious mastitis without medications. When left untreated, it can become infectious and lead to the development of an abscess.

Make sure you get treatment right away if you are experiencing recurrent mastitis. Breast abscess can result from an untreated infection. This condition may require needle aspiration to drain the pus or even surgery. Consult a physician if you have repeated cases of mastitis. It may be a sign of a developing breast tumor.

Prevention of mastitis

-Don't allow your breast to become excessively full. Manually express or pump your milk if your breast still feels full after a feeding. Also,

gentle massage and warm compresses will be helpful if you have a clogged duct.

-Avoid tight clothing. Bras with underwire or tight-fitted tops and swimsuits compress your breast. Such wears can lead to the formation of clogs in milk ducts. Make sure your bra is well-fitted and opt for loose blouses. Also, keep the strap of your bag away from your breast to avoid exerting pressure on it.

-Sudden changes to the nursing schedule can lead to engorgement. Your breasts can become overly full if your baby skips a feeding. Pump the milk to empty your breasts. Gradually reduce the nursing time of the feeding your

baby usually misses. It will help control your milk supply when your baby skips the feeding.

-Consult your lactation consultant when you have issues with breastfeeding. Failure to empty your breasts during feedings can lead to engorgement. However, a lactation consultant will guide and support you to breastfeed successfully.

-Good nutrition and rest can reduce the risk of developing mastitis. Maintain a balanced diet and make out time to relax. Also, increase your fluid intake while breastfeeding.

Supportive measures and complete removal of milk from the inflamed breast can relieve mastitis. The conservative management of this condition is effective if the signs are mild and have existed for less than a day. However, you should start treatment with antibiotics instantly if the symptoms persist after 24 hours or you have flu-like signs.

Continuous breastfeeding when you have mastitis is an effective treatment option. This nursing problem can cause your milk to have a saltier taste as a result of increased levels of sodium and chloride. Though the minerals are good for your baby, the change in taste can put him off. Also, the expressed milk may become clumpy and gelatin-like.

Remember to contact a physician right away if the symptoms are severe or you have a fever.

Also, don't take medications without a doctor's prescription.

CHAPTER 10

THRUSH

Sometimes breastfeeding mothers suffer from nipple and breast pain resulting from thrush. Usually, this condition arises when the nipples are dry or cracked. Thrush is a fungal infection caused by *Candida albicans*, which is a yeast-like organism. This fungus is part of the normal flora of the human digestive system. However, an overgrowth of these organisms can lead to infection.

Candida inhabits the gut, mouth, and vagina due to their preference for warmth and moist environment. You can contact thrush on your areola and nipple from your baby's infected mouth. This yeast infection can make a newborn's mouth sore. Consequently, the baby fuses during nursing.

Also, thrush causes sharp pains at the mother's breasts and nipples during and between feedings. Such discomfort can make nursing mothers dread breastfeeding their babies.

Unfortunately, some of them do quit breastfeeding for fear of the excruciating pain resulting from thrush infection.

Immediate and appropriate treatment is necessary if you have thrush while nursing your baby. Besides, medical support will enable you to breastfeed successfully despite the challenges.

Causes

Your baby can contract thrush from the birth canal during delivery if you have a vaginal yeast infection. Antibiotics taken by mothers during labor or after a c-section or babies after birth can also set off thrush.

Symptoms of oral thrush in breastfeeding infants

Older babies may not show signs of the infection. However, the following are common symptoms.

-Presence of white patches, resembling milk residue, on a baby's gums, tongue or the inside of his cheeks and lips. This white coating may also appear on the roof of his mouth. When wiped with a clean cloth, the white coating remains. Instead, the affected area becomes sore and reddish. Leftover milk appears as a white patch only on your baby's tongue.

-Your baby experiences discomfort and cries during feedings. Pain resulting from the infection can make him slip off the breast.

-Raised diaper rash may appear around the baby's genitals and legs.

Your baby will be fussy during and after nursing if he has oral thrush. The discomfort resulting from the infection can force him to go on a nursing strike. In rare cases, babies may also have an overgrowth of *Candida* without showing visible signs such as white patches on the tongue and inside the mouth.

Such a situation can arise if a mother has taken antibiotics recently. The medication can suppress the non-pathogenic bacteria that protect the body against thrush. However,

Symptoms of thrush in breastfeeding mothers

-Flaky or dry skin on the areola or nipples.

-The skin on the areola or nipples becomes itchy and shiny.

-Burning pain in the nipples.

-Deep shooting pain within the breast(s) which persists through and after feedings.

-Vaginal yeast infection.

Often, the achy feeling starts after a mother has been breastfeeding without experiencing pains.

(Note that the nipple and breast pain occurs without sore lumps). You may feel the pain in both breasts. However, the ache is not the only indication of a thrush infection. While improper latch can also cause nipple pain, the discomfort disappears after feedings.

Treatment of thrush

Both you and your baby need medical attention if either of you has thrush. Cross infection is possible if the mother and newborn do not receive treatment at the same time. Consult a physician for a proper diagnosis if you suspect that you or your baby have a thrush infection.

Your doctor will rule out other causes of breast pain before commencing treatment for thrush.

However, you may not receive medications if you do not have any symptoms while your baby has oral thrush. Your health provider may recommend the following measures if you need treatment.

-Application of antifungal creams such as miconazole on the nipples after each feeding. Make sure you wash your hands thoroughly after rubbing the cream.

-Intake of prescribed antifungal tablets. This treatment option is necessary for severe thrush infection. In such cases, the yeast may have spread to the milk ducts or deeper within the breast.

-Regular intake of painkillers can also reduce the intensity of the pain.

Usually, the antifungal suspension is effective for the treatment of oral thrush in babies. Carefully wash your hands after administering the medication to your baby. Consult your health provider if the symptoms did not improve within one week of the therapy. You can continue breastfeeding while both of you are receiving treatment.

Management of thrush

The following tips will help you deal with thrush infection.

-Try to keep your nipples dry. Gently wipe them after showering and change your breast pad often to prevent the overgrowth *Candida*. The fungus grows well in warm and moist areas.

-Wear a clean bra each day. Make sure your bras are thoroughly washed and dried.

-Treat any fungal infection in you or other members of the family.

-Change towels daily and make sure that members of the family use separate towels.

-Wash your hands thoroughly after changing diapers, visiting the bathroom and application of antifungal creams.

-Clean and sterilize teats, soothers and other things that come in contact with your baby's mouth after use.

-Use a clean damp cloth to wipe your baby's mouth or rinse it if possible with drinking water. It will prevent the yeasts from feeding on the milk residue in his mouth.

-Air your nipples. You can go braless to avoid compressing the nipples.

-Do not freeze any expressed milk if you have thrush. Storing the milk to use it later or after completing treatment will lead to re-infection.

You are likely to have thrush postpartum if you have the infection during pregnancy. The presence of estrogen increases the blood sugar levels, creating a favorable condition for the growth of yeasts. Reducing your intake of carbohydrate-rich foods will help keep the fungus in check.

Increase your fluid intake but avoid sugary drinks. Besides water, herbal teas are an ideal option due to their antioxidant content. Probiotics can facilitate the growth of "friendly bacteria" in the gut. Consume more probiotic yogurts if you or your baby have taken antibiotics after birth or recently.

CHAPTER 11

PAINFUL/ OVERACTIVE LETDOWN

Letdown refers to the release of milk by the producing glands in the breast into the milk ducts. It supports the flow of milk from the breast to your baby. The newborn will only get a portion of the foremilk if there is no release from the glands. A good letdown will enable you to breastfeed your baby properly.

This physiological process occurs more than once during a nursing session. However, most breastfeeding mothers experience only the initial ejection of milk. You can also feel a letdown when you hear your baby cry or think about him.

In both situations, your milk starts to flow when your baby isn't breastfeeding. During a nursing session, letdown occurs after the baby sucks at a breast for a couple of minutes. Besides, it can take place after a few seconds if you have established breastfeeding.

You can feel a tingling sensation during the milk release. You may not experience this feeling in the first few days after birth. However, you will feel the milk ejection when your milk comes in, and you have been nursing for weeks. You may feel the pricking of needles or a squeezing or tingling sensation under your arms and in the direction of your breasts.

You may feel that your breasts are full during a letdown. Also, milk may drip from the other breast that your baby isn't nursing on at the moment. Strong uterine contractions are also common when milk release occurs during the first few days postpartum.

The hot, tingly and rushing feeling diminishes over time in some women. Instead, these moms will experience a warm release as the milk flows through the duct into their nipples.

However, some breastfeeding moms feel nothing during the milk ejection. In such cases, your baby's sucking action will confirm if there is a letdown. Once there is milk ejection, his suction deepens and becomes slow with gradual swallowing movement. Your baby will feel contented after feedings if your letdown is normal. Besides, he will gain weight at an appropriate rate.

Some women have problems with letdown. The breast milk release can be painful or forceful (overactive).

Painful milk ejection

Some breastfeeding mothers experience mild or severe pain when their milk ducts tighten to force milk from the alveoli into their nipples. While some women feel a tingling sensation as the milk flows in the ducts, the movement hurts others. The latter may have a sharp, stabbing pain across their chest during the milk ejection reflex.

Causes of a painful letdown

Extreme pain during milk release may result from the following conditions.

-engorged breasts

-clogged ducts

-production of too much milk or hyperlactation

-mastitis

-thrush

Dealing with letdown pain

Painful milk ejection can discourage you from breastfeeding your baby. This problem may force you to wean him early. The application of moisturizing cream or lotion soothes the breast and eases the discomfort during the letdown process. You can also take a pain reliever such as ibuprofen. However, you need to consult your doctor before taking medications.

Visit a physician immediately you notice symptoms of mastitis or thrush. Breast infections can cause shooting pains during breastfeeding. Medical help will relieve the pain and allow you to enjoy the bonding session with your baby. Also, your baby needs the attention of a pediatrician if he develops oral thrush.

Nurse your baby on one breast at each feeding if the production of too much milk is the cause of the painful letdown. Then switch to the other during the next session and breastfeed him on

168

it alone. This feeding pattern will help train your body to produce less milk.

The breast that is still full at the end of a feeding session will signal to your body to produce less milk. Eventually, your breast milk production will reduce within a few days. With less milk flowing through the ducts, the discomfort during the ejection reflex will lessen.

Try to reduce engorgement if it is the cause of the pain (remedies discussed in Chapter 5). Your breasts will produce only the quantity of milk needed by your baby if they are not engorged. Likewise, the achy feeling during the letdown process will cease.

Overactive letdown

In some breastfeeding mothers, a large quantity of milk is ejected forcefully from the producing glands. Excessive and forceful letdown can inconvenience both baby and mother. It can cause your newborn to cough and choke while breastfeeding. Likewise, you may experience discomfort and pain.

Observe your baby's behavior while nursing to confirm if you have a fast letdown. Your milk ejection is overactive if he chokes and coughs while sucking or pulls off the breast severally. An excessive and forceful letdown occurring early during feeding can cause your baby to swallow air.

Besides, he will consume more foremilk than hindmilk in a gush. The latter is less watery and contains higher levels of fat than the milk at the beginning of a feeding. The breast milk becomes creamier gradually as the baby breastfeeds due to the increased fat content.

Signs of overactive letdown

Besides coughing and choking, the following actions of your baby will suggest forceful ejection of milk.

-Crying while breastfeeding.

-Squeaking or gulping excessively.

-Pulling back at the nipples while breastfeeding.

-Too much spitting up or hiccoughs.

-Milk dribbling from your baby's mouth while feeding.

-Making clicking sounds at the nipples.

These discomforts during feedings indicate an overactive letdown. Also, your baby may develop colic and gassiness as a result of the air he swallowed, and the large quantity of milk consumed. The forceful spray of milk can be distressing for a newborn. Eventually, your baby may refuse to breastfeed.

Tips On Managing Overactive Letdown

172

-Laid back nursing: Changing your feeding position especially when your baby is a few weeks old can deal with forceful milk ejection. You can lie on your back with your baby on top while breastfeeding. This position enables him to pull off the nipple if the milk sprays forcefully during release. Use a burp cloth or diaper to collect the overflow of milk. Then re-attach your baby to the breast when the flow lessens.

-Discontinue feeding during letdown. You can take your baby off the breast immediately the letdown starts. Catch the milk on a clean cloth and continue feeding on the same breast after the milk ejection. Then, your baby can get more of the hindmilk.

-*Clamp down the areola.* Hold the areola between your index and middle fingers. Compressing it with these fingers during the forceful milk release will enable your baby to consume milk at a slow pace.

-*Nurse on one breast at each feeding.* Don't time your baby on the breast. Allow him to feed to his satisfaction. You can nurse on a breast for two subsequent feedings if the other breast is not too engorged. However, you should nurse him frequently. Every two to three hours and even at night will help reduce the intensity of the milk release. Avoid skipping feedings.

-*Express your milk.* Emptying some of your milk before nursing will enable your baby to get

174

more of the rich hindmilk. It will also save him from experiencing the discomfort that results from an overactive letdown. Reducing the milk flow will also help to prevent early weaning. Babies who feel full after feeding on the breast milk in a gush are likely to wean early.

The measures discussed above can help both newborns and older babies to manage overactive letdown. Besides, it is necessary to treat hyperlactation if the forceful milk ejection comes with excessive supply.

Don't introduce bottle-feeding to a baby experiencing discomfort from intense milk flow. The baby may prefer the artificial nipple which will be more comfortable to suck on than

the breast. Such a situation can lead to nipple
eventually, breast rejection.

Slow Letdown

Besides painful/overactive milk ejection, some
breastfeeding mothers experience slow letdown
reflex. Such a situation can frustrate a hungry
baby. He may start crying or bite your nipple if
there is a delay in the milk release. Also, pain
accompanies this nursing problem.

Slow milk ejection can result from stress,
exhaustion, smoking, and alcohol intake. Gentle
massaging, use of warm compresses, and
pumping your breast milk can help improve the

condition. Also, increase your fluid intake. Eat healthy and balance meals. Try to avoid alcohol and smoking.

CHAPTER 12

HYPERLACTATION

Low milk supply is one of the common breastfeeding issues. However, some nursing mothers experience abundant production of breast milk. The oversupply of milk may not seem to be a problem for many, but it can affect breastfeeding negatively.

You may produce more milk than your baby requires in the first six weeks of breastfeeding. However, a plentiful milk supply that persists after this period is an indication of hyperlactation. Women who are experiencing an oversupply of milk will notice that their milk often soaks their breast pads and clothes. It also sprays a lot.

Hyperlactation can cause forceful ejection of milk, which can make your baby choke. Besides, he may become fussy during feedings and experience constant stomach discomfort.

Symptoms of hyperlactation

Oversupply of breast milk is a common breastfeeding problem during the first three months postpartum. Early detection of this condition can help you to improve your baby's breastfeeding experience.

Mother's symptoms

-Constant feeling of engorgement in both breasts.

-Plugged ducts, which may result in mastitis develops.

-Pain may accompany forceful milk ejection.

-Excessive leaking of milk. Your breast milk may leak between feedings and from the other breast while nursing your baby.

-Your milk sprays when it leaks. Also, spraying of milk is likely to occur at the beginning of feedings if your baby slips off the breast while feeding

A mother may start experiencing these symptoms in the first week after birth. In some cases, the signs begin to manifest within the first two or three weeks postpartum. Your milk supply may become normal on its own without treatment during the first three months after birth. However, hyperlactation may persist until the fifth month after birth.

Baby's symptoms

-Your baby finds it difficult to maintain a good latch while nursing and may slip off the breast when the letdown occurs.

-He may clamp down on your nipple while feeding, especially after sucking for about five to ten minutes.

-He becomes fussy during feedings.

-During nursing, the infant may gulp, gag, and sputter.

-Your baby often spits up milk excessively after feeding. This symptom of hyperlactation may be mistaken for reflux.

182

-Your baby prefers frequent and short feedings as he feels full so fast and stops nursing.

-Your baby may pass gas frequently due to air trapped during nursing and foremilk/hindmilk imbalance.

-Your baby consumes much foremilk which results in massive, explosive, frothy or watery green stools.

-Your baby may have a high and rapid weight gain if he consumes large quantities of milk. However, his weight gain may be lower than average if he can't nurse effectively.

Due to the oversupply of breast milk, your baby gets filled up quickly on the watery foremilk that is rich in lactose. He may stop nursing without draining the hindmilk with higher fat content which is creamy. The excessive lactose in the baby's intestines will result in colic-like symptoms. These signs include discomfort, gassiness, and watery or foamy green stools.

Over time, a small amount of blood may appear in your baby's stools. This occurrence results from the irritation of the intestines' lining by the accumulated undigested lactose. Most of the time, foremilk/hindmilk imbalance in babies is mistaken for lactose intolerance or food allergies.

Causes of hyperlactation

During pregnancy, your body prepares for milk production. When you put to bed, your hormone signals to your body to start supplying breast milk. However, while some mothers produce too little milk, others make more than their babies need. Even when their milk supply has established, these moms can still experience overabundance production of milk. The following factors can cause hyperlactation in nursing mothers.

Possession of above-average number of alveoli

Breast milk is stored temporarily in the milk-producing glands, alveoli, before the draining of the breasts. Most women have about 100,000 alveoli in each breast. However, women that have around 300,000 alveoli are likely to experience hyperlactation.

Pumping of the breasts

How often and the quantity of milk removed from the breasts determines how much milk your body produces. Once you have established breastfeeding, your body adjusts to the nursing routine. It can figure out the quantity of milk your baby needs during the feeding sessions.

In most women, it takes up to three months for the body to adjust to the needs of the baby. However, the timing may differ between pregnancies and from one breastfeeding mom to another.

Pumping can cause your body to produce too much milk. When you pump more than the quantity you baby needs at a feeding, you are indirectly forcing your body to supply more milk. Your mammary glands notice the increase in the quantity of milk drained from the breasts and will increase its production to satisfy the demand. However, they cannot differentiate suction by a pump from the emptying of the breasts by the baby during a nursing session.

You may need to pump milk for your baby if you are a working mom. It is crucial that you pump only the quantity your baby takes at a

187

feeding to avoid hyperlactation. Don't give your body the notion that your baby's appetite has increased by pumping excessively.

Pumping isn't a good option when you are already experiencing an oversupply of milk. It will signal your body to produce more milk since you are still taking out more milk than your baby needs at each feeding.

Feeding techniques

Your breastfeeding tactics can subject your body to an oversupply of milk. You may have followed the counsel of concerned friends and family members. They may advise you to feed on both breasts at each feeding. Some people may recommend that you pump a full breast before nursing to make it softer and easy for your baby to grip. These techniques may lead to an oversupply of breast milk.

Your baby may also stimulate your body to produce more milk if he often feeds on one breast continuously. This situation causes an oversupply in one breast (the preferred side) since the baby feeds on it consistently and longer than the other.

Ideally, allow your baby to empty one breast completely during a feeding before you put him on the second side. Put him first on the opposite breast at the next session. Switch to the first side again when he finished sucking the breast. This approach will help control your supply of breast milk. Besides, it will enable your baby to have an excellent foremilk-hindmilk balance at each feeding.

Hormonal imbalance

Hyperlactation may result from changes in your hormones. A medical examination of the pituitary gland can help determine problems that can lead to hormonal imbalance. Hormones control milk production after birth.

However, individuals react differently to these hormones. You may experience hyperlactation if your body responds readily to these hormones. After some time, the frequency and effective draining of the breasts take over the regulation of milk supply.

The intake of certain drugs that cause hormonal imbalance can also lead to an oversupply of breast milk. Always consult a physician before taking any medication when nursing a baby.

Overproduction of breast milk may also occur as a result of your genetic make-up. No two individuals are the same. If you produce a lot of milk, it may not be as a result of your actions or your baby's. Your body functions may be responsible for this breastfeeding challenge.

Dealing With An Oversupply Of Breast Milk

The overproduction of breast milk poses a problem in breastfeeding. Many mothers experience this challenge before their bodies start regulating milk production. In most cases, the milk supply normalizes when the baby's demand start controlling the quantity of milk produced.

Besides, the condition may persist when your body is controlling milk production. Several factors may cause hyperlactation during this period. It is important to consider the age of your baby and the causes of the oversupply before you try to regulate your milk supply.

Managing postpartum oversupply of breast milk

It is not advisable to reduce milk supply in the first few months after birth. During this period, hormones regulate the production of breast milk. Correcting an early oversupply may lead to a decrease in milk production later.

You can manage the situation until you have established breastfeeding. Here are tips that tips will help you to handle oversupply of milk in the early months after birth.

Reverse pressure softening

Gently massage your breasts with your fingers before feedings if they are engorged. Massaging will soften the breasts and facilitate better latching. Unlike pumping, manipulating the engorged breasts with your fingers does not encourage the overproduction of milk. However, it stimulates a letdown which helps to reduce the pressure in the breast.

Unlatch your baby during letdowns

An oversupply of milk can lead to forceful milk ejections. Take your baby off the breast when the initial letdown occurs. You can collect the milk that flows out in a clean bottle (if you want to save it) or towel. Put your baby on the breast again when the pressure of the milk flow reduces.

Change feeding position

During feedings, incline your baby at an angle that will force the milk to flow upwards. Uphill nursing can help control the forceful flow of milk. You can opt for any position that is comfortable for you and the baby. Breastfeed your baby while lying on your side. Use a clean towel to collect the dripping milk. You can also nurse your baby while he sits and faces you. However, you may need to tilt his head back a little.

Don't pump if possible

Pumping milk to feed the baby in your absence may seem to be a good idea. However, it can encourage the overproduction of breast milk. It is better to pump when you have established breastfeeding.

Dealing with hyperlactation

An oversupply of milk may persist a few months after birth. Consult a lactation consultant to help you reduce your milk supply. You may try the suggestions below under the supervision of the professional.

Cabbage leaf compresses

This remedy has been in use for ages. Besides relieving breast engorgement, placing cabbage leaves in your bra can reduce milk supply. Apply chilled and washed cabbage leaves to your breasts between feedings. However, you should use the vegetables for short periods as they can suppress milk production.

Adopt block feeding

Nurse your baby on only one breast for a few feedings (two to four) in a row before switching to the second breast. While using one breast for block feeding, hand express some milk from the other if it is uncomfortably engorged. Emptying it a bit will relieve pressure and reduce the risk of clogged ducts.

Alternatively, pump both breasts to empty the accumulated milk before you start the block feeding immediately. Draining the "milk lakes" will help readjust your milk production. However, don't pump after nursing to avoid a further increase in your milk supply. Stop pumping milk to feed your baby when separated until your baby's demand start regulating your milk production.

Use the minimum setting when using the pump machine to drain your breast. A gentle suction will stimulate the breast, less.

Medications

Certain medicines can reduce breast milk production. However, such a situation is a side effect of using the medications. Consequently, nursing mothers should consult physicians before using hormonal contraceptives and other medicines that can inhibit milk supply.

Besides, these medications can have other adverse effects on the body. It is advisable to use medicines to regulate your milk supply only when recommended by a doctor and if you have exhausted other options.

Herbs

The medicinal plant, sage, can reduce milk production. However, it should be used with caution as the herb can stop lactation.

Breastfeeding your baby when he is less hungry will help control your milk flow if you are experiencing an oversupply. Also, treat mastitis or blocked ducts if you have developed these conditions before trying to control the oversupply.

Donate your milk

Alternatively, you can maintain the oversupply and donate your milk to a human milk bank. Donated breast milk is useful for the nourishment of newborns in the Intensive Care Unit (ICU).

Hyperlactation can interfere with breastfeeding. It can cause a baby to reject the breasts. Effective management of an oversupply of milk will enable mother and baby to have a pleasurable breastfeeding experience. However, you should avoid unverified practices.

Do not bind your breasts as it can lead to plugged ducts. Limiting the nursing time or feeding your baby on a schedule can reduce his milk intake. It can also lead to low milk production.

CHAPTER 13

LEAKING BREASTS

Mia, a first-time mom, noticed that her milk leaks mostly in the mornings and sometimes from one breast during feedings. She also experienced the same situation at times from both breasts when she wasn't nursing her baby, even at nights. She was upset at the development. Mia consulted a lactation professional who gave the tips that enabled her to manage the condition.

Many women find it difficult to keep their nursing tops dry while breastfeeding. Leaking breasts may be frustrating, but it indicates that the mammary glands are functioning well. Some moms may leak milk only during the first few weeks of breastfeeding their babies. However, the condition may persist for months.

It is normal for your breasts to leak in the early weeks of breastfeeding. They may spray milk when they are full, especially in the mornings and during feedings. Moreover, women who produce too much milk are likely to experience leaking breasts.

Leaking of milk relieves the feeling of fullness in the breasts. It can also prevent engorgement and clogging of milk ducts since the milk leaks when the ducts are overfill. While some nursing moms never leak, others experience the condition for months or throughout the breastfeeding period.

Leaking breasts occurs naturally in nursing moms. This condition is common in the first few weeks after birth. However, your milk production will adjust to your baby's demand during the first 6 to 10 weeks after delivery. The time it takes for the quantity of milk the baby consumes to regulate milk supply differs among individuals.

Once you have established breastfeeding, your milk may occasionally spray during letdowns, while pumping or when you skip a feeding. However, excessive leaking persists in some moms. Such condition is common with women that are experiencing an oversupply of milk.

Why do breasts leak?

Oxytocin, a hormone that stimulates milk letdown, is responsible for leaking breasts. Due to the milk ejection reflex, your milk can leak from the other breast while you breastfeed your baby. Your baby's suction initiates milk ejection.

Your breasts may also spray milk or leak when you experience unexpected letdowns. Some mothers may leak milk when they think of their babies or hear them cry. You may also experience an overflow of milk when your breasts are full. Such leaking usually occurs in the mornings and during feedings when the milk supply is at its peak.

Relaxation and warmth can also stimulate milk flow. Consequently, your breasts may leak during a shower or when you are in a heated room. Overproduction of breast milk can also lead to spraying of milk during forceful letdowns.

Besides, excessive breast leaking may result from sleep deprivation, chronic fatigue, and nervousness. In such cases, affected breastfeeding mothers should consume a balanced diet and get enough sleep. Consulting a lactation professional on their emotional state will also help.

Dealing with leaking breasts

Spraying of milk from the breasts can be embarrassing. However, it is a sign that your body is functioning properly to provide nourishment for your baby. The following tips will help you manage the spraying of milk from the breasts.

Frequent nursing

Most women experience an oversupply in the first few weeks after birth. Nurse your baby often during this period to prevent an overflow when your breasts are full. The more frequent you nurse your baby; the less likely your breasts are to leak. Avoid long intervals between feeding sessions.

Make sure that your baby makes a good latch on the breasts during feedings. You will produce the quantity of milk required by your baby at each feeding when you have established breastfeeding.

Express milk to relieve pressure

Breastfeeding more often can help prevent your breasts from becoming too full. Express enough milk to make you comfortable if your baby is away from you or not ready to nurse when your breasts are overfill. Draining the breasts when you feel that fullness will help prevent leaks. You can feed your baby the expressed milk after he has nursed on the breasts.

Do not remove so much milk to provoke an increase in your milk supply. However, you may develop mastitis or plugged duct if you don't breastfeed or pump when your breasts are full.

Control the letdowns

Many women experience a tingly sensation before milk ejection occurs. Gently apply pressure to your breasts when you experience such feelings to prevent your milk from leaking.

209

You can press your thumbs or the base of your palms over your nipples.

Besides, pressing your forearms firmly into your breasts while cupping your chin with both hands when you feel that your milk is about to drip may be helpful. This posture is more effective than other control methods if your elbows are supported on a table while sitting.

You can also cross your arms over your chest to stop the unexpected flow of milk. However, avoid much pressure on full breasts. It can encourage the development of mastitis.

Use washable nursing pads

Some women do not experience the tingling feeling that precedes a letdown. Such individuals need to prepare for the leakages to avoid embarrassment. Place a breast pad in your nursing bra to soak up the milk.

Cloth nursing pads are preferable. You can cut up cloth diapers to improvise breast pads. However, make sure you change them often. They can breed bacteria when damp. Carry extra nursing pads when you are out. Changing them often will keep your nipples dry.

Avoid nursing pads with plastic lining. They can trap moisture on the areola while keeping your cloth dry. The dampness can lead to nipple soreness. It can also encourage the development of infections such as thrush.

Use a clean towel or diaper

During the breastfeeding sessions, soak up the milk that leaks from the other breast with a clean cloth. Using a diaper or towel while nursing at home will help save your breast pads for outings. You can also collect the leaking milk and save it for later use.

Place a clean bath towel on your bed. It will soak up leaked milk and protect the bed sheet from stains. Nursing your baby before you go to bed at night can also minimize leaking.

Camouflage clothing

Wear clothes that can hide milk stains. Prints are an ideal option. Pack an extra top for outings. It can save the day. Besides, you can carry a sweater or jacket that you can easily put on if your breasts start leaking.

Nursing moms don't wish to experience wet and sticky breasts. Such a situation can make you uncomfortable especially if the leaking is excessive. Planning will enable you to deal with an overflow of milk when your breasts are full. If you are using breast shields to correct inverted nipples switch to nipple shields.

Breast shells or shields are plastic cups. When worn over the breasts, they press firmly on them to push the nipples out through the openings. They may stimulate the breasts to leak milk.

Despite the leaking breasts, you can still nurse your baby. The condition boosts your confidence in your ability to breastfeed. You have enough milk to provide natural nourishment for your baby. Certainly, you will enjoy a pleasurable breastfeeding experience with your baby once the leaking subsides.

CHAPTER 14

LOW MILK SUPPLY

Sometimes you may find breastfeeding difficult and confusing, especially if you are a first-time mom. Though a natural act, you need to learn the proper latch technique and determine the nursing positions that are suitable for your baby.

Despite your willingness to breastfeed successfully, you may worry if you are producing enough milk to satisfy him. You may think that your supply is low if milk no longer leaks from your nipples or your breasts no longer feel full. An increase in your baby's feeding demand may lead to these changes.

Normally, your breasts will no longer feel full when your baby is about two months old. Due to growth, your baby may need to nurse often. He drains more milk with longer and frequent feedings than usual. This nursing pattern will not lower your milk supply. Instead, it will help you to build and maintain it.

Besides the adjustment of the body to satisfy a baby's nursing requirement, some mothers experience low milk supply. You need to check out whether your baby consumes more milk than usual or your supply is low. The latter condition can limit exclusive breastfeeding. Cases of inadequate milk production can be corrected to prevent your baby from malnutrition.

Your baby may lose or not gain weight if he isn't getting enough milk regularly. This condition can hinder both mental and physical development. Visit your baby's pediatrician if you notice that the infant requires more milk than the quantity he gets.

The doctor can rule out other health issues associated with poor weight gain. Besides, other nursing problems such as breast engorgement, sore nipples, and a nursing strike can affect the quantity of milk your baby gets.

Mothers experiencing low milk supply may become frustrated at their inability to satisfy their babies' feeding demand. However, nursing for longer periods and frequently can boost milk supply. You may need to correct your baby's latch or even pump to make sure that he gets enough milk.

Causes of low milk supply

A baby's inability to satisfy his nursing demand may result from either the production or delivery of the breast milk. Inadequate production of breast milk is rare as most mothers produce more milk than their babies require.

However, some factors such as previous breast surgery, hormonal and physical conditions, maternal obesity, medications, and premature birth can make a mother susceptible to low milk supply.

Your milk supply may temporarily reduce if you don't nurse your baby often. Besides, waiting for long before starting breastfeeding or supplementing your baby's feeding can lessen your milk supply. A poor latch can also limit the quantity of milk your baby gets during nursing. Correcting an improper latch technique will be helpful in this case.

The causes of low milk supply may either result from a mother or her baby. However, identifying these factors will help you to manage the condition appropriately and still breastfeed your baby.

Problems linked to mothers

Nursing issues

Conditions such as cracked nipples, clogged ducts, engorgement, mastitis, and thrush can interfere with milk supply. Treat these problems once they develop to maintain a pleasurable breastfeeding experience. Also, you need to seek the guidance of a lactation consultant if you have inverted or flat nipples to make sure that your baby gets enough milk.

Maternal obesity

Some obese mothers can satisfy their babies' nursing requirements. However, there are others with the same condition that experience low milk supply. Obesity can delay milk production in breastfeeding mothers.

Medications

Contraceptives that contain estrogen (or a combination of progesterone and estrogen) can also reduce milk production. Progestin-only birth control methods such as the implant, mini-pills, and Mirena IUD are ideal for nursing mothers. These options can't interfere with the quantity of breast milk you produce. However, you need to consult your health provider for a birth control method that suits you most.

Most cold and allergy medications contain pseudoephedrine, which can lower breast milk production. Avoid such medications in the early weeks of breastfeeding when the milk supply isn't well-established. However, a dosage later may not affect your milk production.

Hormonal disorder

Conditions associated with hormones such as thyroid imbalance can affect breast milk supply negatively. The thyroid aids the regulation of oxytocin and prolactin. Low thyroid will affect this function and lead to a decrease in the amount of milk produced.

Insufficient supply of blood to the pituitary (Sheehan's Syndrome) due to excessive blood loss during childbirth can affect breastfeeding. This condition deprives the gland of oxygen needed for effective functioning. The disorder results in the inability of the pituitary gland to produce hormones such as prolactin which is responsible for breast milk production.

Physical conditions

Pregnancy-induced blood pressure, insulin-dependent diabetes, and anemia can affect milk production. Breast surgery, particularly reduction procedures can increase the risk of low milk supply. Medications and dietary changes are crucial in the treatment of these conditions.

Intake of iron supplements and adjustments to your diet are helpful in the treatment of iron-deficiency anemia. This condition, which results from increased blood requirements during pregnancy and blood loss via menstruation, can lower milk production.

Consumption of anti-lactogenic herbs and spices

Intake of some herbs and spices can lower milk supply. Sage, parsley, thyme, oregano, and peppermint can reduce milk supply in some mothers, especially when consumed in large quantities. Dietary adjustment to eliminate non-lactogenic foods can help improve your milk production. However, mothers who are not experiencing difficulties in maintaining their milk supply may not be affected by these spices and herbs.

Unhealthy habits

Smoking can lower milk supply in some mothers. However, some mothers who smoke cigarette still nurse their babies successfully. Intake of nicotine and alcohol can also have the same effect.

Low milk production can also result from the retention of fragments of the placenta, especially after a Caesarean section.

Issues related to babies

Premature birth

Babies born before the due date are usually fragile and require more care and time to grow. Such infants have under-developed suck reflex. Eventually, they will have difficulty breastfeeding since they can't suck and swallow effectively. Failure to empty the breasts can lower the milk supply.

Congenital malformations

A baby with badly formed mouthparts such as cleft-palette or cleft-lip will find it difficult to drain milk from the breasts. These malformations prevent a close up around the nipple and consequently milk from getting to the baby.

Mouth issues

Conditions such as a tongue tie and bubble or high palette can limit the quantity of milk that your baby gets from the breasts.

Neurological problems

Disordered breathing, sucking or swallowing reflex can prevent a baby from nursing effectively. An infant with such an issue requires assistance during feedings to satisfy his nursing demands. Also, medical treatment can help to correct the condition.

Down syndrome

Due to low muscle tone, breastfeeding a baby with Down syndrome can be challenging. This condition also reduces the muscle strength of lips and tongues of affected babies. Such infants nurse poorly and may experience low weight gain. During breastfeeding sessions, good head support can facilitate their sucking ability. However, top-up feeds using pumped breast milk can help.

Besides, colicky behavior may result from Gastro-esophageal reflux disease (GERD). This condition can prevent your baby from getting enough milk from the breasts during feedings. Under the guidance of a lactation professional, a mother can overcome the baby's problems that contribute to low milk supply.

You need to consult your physician if you suspect that you have a persistent low milk supply. Your healthcare provider will conduct diagnostic tests to determine the cause of the chronic condition and provide appropriate treatment.

Guidance from lactation and health professionals, dietary and lifestyle changes, and medical treatment can resolve conditions that cause low milk production in nursing mothers. However, the issue of placenta retention can resolve weeks after birth.

How to improve milk supply

Milk removal is vital in maintaining or increasing milk supply. Frequent nursing and expression of breast milk (manually or using an electric pump) can empty your breasts and encourage the production of more milk.

You will have to express your milk to build the supply if your baby is premature or have special needs. Fragile infants aren't strong enough to suck effectively. Feeding them with expressed milk resolves the situation.

The following tips will help if you are not producing enough milk for your baby.

-Nurse your baby often. Frequent breastfeeding encourages your body to make more milk. Allow him to nurse until he is satisfied.

-Position your baby well and make sure he makes a good latch. Make sure your baby is swallowing when he starts nursing.

-Pump your breasts between feedings and use the expressed milk to top up feedings. The pumping action stimulates the production of more milk. Also, try to pump your breasts each time you skip a feeding. It will help maintain your milk supply.

-Offer your baby both breasts at each nursing session. Switch him to the second breast when his sucking and swallowing slows down.

-Stop using a pacifier. You can encourage your baby to suck for comfort at the breast. The suction will stimulate your body to produce more milk.

-Avoid supplementing your baby's feedings. Introducing formula or solid food to your baby before six months of age can make him lose interest in breastfeeding. Consequently, his preference for formula or solid food can lead to a decrease in your milk production. Try feeding him with a spoon, dropper or cup if his pediatrician suggests supplementing breastfeeding for medical reasons.

-Consume lactogenic foods, beverages, and herbs to increase your milk production. However, you need to consult your doctor about the safety of the herbs you use while breastfeeding.

-Supplements and lactation enhancing medications can also help boost your milk supply. However, you need to consult your physician before taking any medication.

Seek the help of a physician if you still suspect that your milk supply is low. Satisfying your baby's nursing requirement is crucial for his health, growth, and development.

Is your baby getting sufficient milk?

The size of the breast doesn't determine the quantity of milk produced. Each nipple has an average of 9 holes while some have more. The milk sprays out from these holes when the baby sucks. Babies instinctively draw milk from the breasts. Their sucking and swallowing action can control the flow of breast milk.

At the initial stage of feeding, your baby sucks faster on the breast to stimulate the flow of milk. The sucking rhythm becomes slower when you let down until the baby feels satisfied. Babies normally breathe while sucking on the breast. An infant can pause while nursing with the breast still in his mouth if he is not full. Your baby will only let go of the breast when he is satisfied and not when he empties it.

Your baby's diapers and growth pattern determines whether he is getting enough milk. Babies gain weight when they are breastfeeding well. From five days to two months of life, most babies have 3 to 4 bowel movements daily. It may become fewer after eight weeks of age as the baby develops a pattern. However, babies have 5 to 6 sopping wet diapers every 24 hours at this age. The pattern of the yellow bowel movement and a good weight gain shows that your baby draws sufficient milk from the breasts.

The following are signs that your baby obtains enough milk from the breast.

-Your baby nurses often, at least every 2-3 hours. Make sure your baby has a minimum of eight feedings a day.

-He appears satisfied after each feeding.

-He gains weight appropriately depending on his age. Your baby should regain his birth age after two weeks of birth.

236

-Your breasts feel softer and no longer after nursing your baby.

-Most babies have at least three bowel movements in the first four weeks of life. The stools may become fewer after two months of age. Your baby may go a day or two without bowel movement as he grows older than when younger.

-Your baby passes enough pale yellow or clear urine. Wetting five to six disposables or seven to eight cloth diapers is an indication that he gets enough milk. A wet disposable is slightly heavier than a dry one. However, wet diapers are inconclusive in determining whether a baby obtains sufficient breast milk.

237

You can hear your baby swallowing if he drains milk effectively from the breasts. However, weight gain and bowel movement are excellent ways of determining whether your baby gets enough milk.

CHAPTER 15

BREAST PREFERENCE

Preferring a breast to the other is a common nursing problem, especially in newborns. Your baby may pull away, fuss or refuse to suck one of your breasts when you try to nurse him on it.

A newborn will still get enough milk if he feeds only on one breast. The preferred breast produces more milk the more your baby sucks it than the other. You may allow your baby to continue nursing on one breast alone. Breastfeeding on demand will enable him to obtain enough milk from only one breast.

You may pump the less desired breast or allow it to dry up if your baby prefers one-sided breastfeeding. However, many mothers will not choose the second option until they wean their babies. In such a situation, you can find solutions to this problem.

Causes of breast preference

Differences are likely to exist between a woman's breasts. Their sizes, the milk flow or even the quantity of milk produced may not be the same. These differences may contribute to one-sided breastfeeding in infants. The conditions below can lead to breast preference in babies.

-Latching difficulty can cause a newborn to reject a breast. Your baby may find it hard to latch on to your breast if it is engorged or there is a difference in the nipples. Such variation may result from the presence of hair or a mole on one of the nipples.

-Variation in milk flow. Your baby may prefer the breast with a faster flow. Consistent nursing

on a particular breast can lead to low milk supply in the abandoned breast. This situation may arise when you forget to switch your baby to the other breast during feedings. Nursing only on the preferred breast may also lead to low milk supply on the other breast.

An older baby is likely to reject the breast that has a low milk supply. You need to consult a physician or lactation professional if you notice that one of your breasts is producing less milk than the other. Physical difference such as surgery in one breast or injury can also lead to lower milk flow. Besides, previous breast cancer treatment or milk ducts filled with cancerous cells can cause the same problem.

-*Saltier taste*. An infant may reject a particular breast if it produces milk with a different taste. Low milk supply can cause a breast to produce saltier milk than the other. Pumping the affected breast can stimulate an increase in milk supply.

Mastitis can also cause breast milk to have a saltier taste by increasing its sodium content. Consequently, if one of your breasts is affected by mastitis, your baby may reject it due to the difference in the taste of its milk.

-*Need for comfort*. Your baby may develop a sudden preference for one breast if nursing on the other side is uncomfortable or painful. Ear infection, blocked nostril or even a sore inside the mouth can cause pain to a baby during breastfeeding. The infant may feel more comfortable when held on a particular side. Eventually, the baby will develop a preference for the breast on that side.

Check your baby for something that might be hurting him if he feels more relaxed on one side than the other. Besides, a tender spot resulting from a recent immunization may be the cause of the sudden one-sided breastfeeding preference.

A mom may also feel at ease nursing from one side consistently. Such a habit can encourage a baby to prefer one breast to the other. Try various breastfeeding positions to find one that will be comfortable for you to nurse on both breasts (Read more about breastfeeding positions in Chapter Two of this book).

-*Birth trauma*. Stiff neck resulting from strain during birth can cause newborns to prefer nursing on one side than the other. Contact your health provider to if you suspect that your baby is suffering from birth injuries. A physical examination will be an ideal option.

Consult a physician if low milk supply persists after pumping, and your baby rejects the affected breast. The presence of cancerous cells may be the cause of the problem.

Dealing with breast preference

You can successfully breastfeed your baby on only one breast and allow the less preferred one to dry up. However, many moms do not want to look lopsided. The following tips will help to correct one-sided breastfeeding.

-Persistently persuade your baby to suck the less desired breast. Nurse him first on it when he is very hungry or immediately he wakes up and is still sleepy. You can place him in the same position as when nursing on the preferred breast.

Alternatively, you can start the nursing session on the desired side. Then, gently move your baby to the less preferred breast immediately let down occurs without changing the nursing position. Football hold and cradle position can do the trick.

-Nurse your baby on the less preferred breast while bouncing, swaying or rocking him. You can also breastfeed while walking. The motion can calm your baby and encourage him to feed on the less desired breast.

-Try various breastfeeding positions. Nursing while lying down may solve the problem. However, don't force him to feed on the less preferred breast as it might result in a nursing strike.

-Use a nipple shield on the less desired breast if its nipple is different from the preferred side.

-Your baby may refuse to nurse if the milk ejection is forceful or too slow. Express some milk from the breast with forceful letdown before nursing your baby. It will decrease the milk flow and prevent your baby from choking. Conversely, you can hasten the milk flow by compressing the breast while nursing.

-Try to increase the milk supply of the less preferred breast if it is low. Gently massage it to prevent the formation of plugs in the milk ducts and boost the milk supply. Pumping the breast for at least 5-10 minutes after each feeding can also help to maintain the supply.

You may store the expressed milk and use it to supplement your baby's feedings. Pumping can

248

also help to even out the variation between the sizes of the breasts.

Finding out the cause of your baby's breast preference will help solve this nursing problem. Have a pediatrician conduct a physical examination on the infant to check for any birth injury. You can also consult your physician to find out if you have breast problems.

Successful breastfeeding is possible from only a breast

Over time, most babies will take the less preferred breast. However, you can nurse your baby only on one breast if you aren't bothered about being lopsided. Your baby's preference for a breast will not be a problem if he gets enough milk from it. Nurse him on demand to maintain the milk supply.

You may pump the less desired breast to retain its milk supply if you are trying to get your baby to nurse on it again. However, you may allow it to dry up if you have decided to nurse only on the preferred side. You can use breast pads to improve its size but the difference in the sizes of the two breasts will even out after weaning your baby.

CHAPTER 16

NURSING STRIKE

Claire is a mother of three. She had successfully breastfed her two older kids. After three months of nursing her third child, the baby suddenly stopped breastfeeding. When her baby refused to nurse despite the hunger cues during the first feeding that fateful day, she was confused.

She realized that something was wrong when the baby behaved in the same manner during the subsequent feedings. She knew her baby was too young to wean on his own. Claire consulted her baby's pediatrician right away. The physician diagnosed the baby with an ear infection which resulted in his refusal to nurse.

A nursing strike is an abrupt refusal of the breast by babies who had happily nursed previously for some months. Something may be wrong if your baby refuses to breastfeed when you aren't weaning him. A baby who abruptly stops nursing may be sick or unhappy.

Though babies can wean on their own, they do so gradually. Self-weaning isn't sudden and hardly occurs before six months of age. Older babies can wean by themselves, but the weaning process cannot make them miserable. The refusal to breastfeed can make your baby unhappy. It can also be frustrating to mother. You may worry about your baby's nourishment if he hasn't started taking solid foods.

This condition can last for a few days or a week. In some cases, it may persist for over a week. A medical examination will help to detect the cause of the sudden breast refusal. You can encourage your baby to breastfeed again if he is experiencing a nursing strike. Though it may take some days, you need to be determined and patient. However, some mothers whose babies are older than six months may opt to wean them during a nursing strike.

Your breasts may become uncomfortably full if your baby skips feedings. You need to express the milk to avoid engorgement, development of mastitis and plugged ducts. Draining your breasts can help you to stay comfortable. Besides, you can use the expressed milk to feed your baby if he continues to refuse the breasts.

Use a dropper, cup or syringe to feed him to avoid nipple confusion. It will also make it easier to get him back to the breasts. Use a hospital-grade electric pump to express your milk as often as your baby used to nurse if you can't do it manually. Expressing your milk will also help to maintain its supply.

Causes of a nursing strike

Several factors can cause abrupt refusal of the breast in babies.

Sickness

Your baby may find it difficult to breathe while nursing if he has a stuffy nose. Unclogging the congested nose can ease the condition. You can use a humidifier, saline drops or nasal aspirator. Consult your health provider on how to use these methods to unclog a stuffy nose. Your physician may also recommend medications that can minimize mucus production.

Mouth pain resulting from cold sores or infections such as thrush can make breastfeeding uncomfortable. Your baby may refuse the breast if it is painful to breastfeed. He may prefer feeding from bottles since it requires less mouth movement and effort to drain the milk. This preference may lead to nipple confusion. Consequently, it is vital to feed your baby the expressed milk with a cup during a nursing strike.

An ear infection can also cause your baby to refuse the breast. He may feel uncomfortable lying on his infected ear to nurse. Change the nursing position to avoid pressure on that ear. You may try the football hold or breastfeed him in an upright position.

Teething

Your baby may experience discomfort as he grows his first teeth. Mouth pain resulting from teething can force your baby to start a nursing strike. However, some babies may nurse more often while teething.

Low milk supply

A slow letdown or reduced milk supply can force your baby to reject the breasts. The overuse of pacifiers or bottles and long intervals between feedings can lower your milk supply. Your baby's suction stimulates your body to produce more milk. However, when your milk supply is low, your baby will not nurse long on your breasts. Eventually, he may go on a nursing strike when the supply didn't increase.

Disrupted nursing routine

Your baby may refuse to nurse if he has skipped his feedings consistently. Such disruption in the nursing schedule may arise if a mother is sick or separated from her baby for a long period. Your baby may not be willing to resume nursing if you leave him for a prolonged period, say a weekend.

Reaction to stress

Your baby's abrupt refusal of the breast may be a response to negative stimuli. Your overreaction, when bitten by your baby during nursing, can startle him. Consequently, he may be scared to breastfeed if you have beaten him.

Stress affecting a mother such as grief or divorce can cause a baby to refuse breasts. A change in environment and disturbances from siblings during feeding sessions may lead to a nursing strike.

Change in breast milk's taste

The intake of a drug or vitamin can cause a change in the taste of your milk. Hormonal changes resulting from your menstrual period or pregnancy can also have the same effect. Use of perfumed ointments or creams or a change of toiletries can make you smell differently to your baby. It is ideal to use the tasteless and odorless lanolin formulated for breastfeeding mothers while nursing.

Besides, excessive caffeine or certain foods such as dairy products can encourage a nursing strike. The breast infection, mastitis, can also make your milk taste salty. The sodium levels in your milk may increase if your breast milk supply decreases following this infection. However, the salty taste is not a permanent change.

Dealing with a nursing strike

The nursing strike may last for a few days or longer. Forcing your baby to breastfeed during this period may frustrate him. Consequently, he may develop negative feelings about nursing. You need to be persistent and patient while encouraging him to return to the breast.

Try feeding your baby with the expressed milk if he still refuses the breasts. It is preferable to feed your baby the expressed milk in a sippy cup or use a dropper or spoon. Express your milk manually or use a pump as often as your baby used to nurse. Emptying your breasts will prevent engorgement and plugged ducts. It will also maintain your milk supply.

However, these tips will help you to overcome nursing strike.

Consult your baby's pediatrician to rule out medical conditions (thrush or ear infection) that may lead to a nursing strike. Also, seek advice on alternative feeding if your baby still refuses to nurse.

Nurse your baby in a quiet environment to avoid distractions. A dark or dimly lit room will be ideal. Avoid sounds from television or radio.

However, some low volume of soothing music may be helpful. Babies don't settle down to nurse when they are distracted. Older infants (6-9 months) are most affected since they have become aware of their surroundings. They will play when you put them on the breast to feed.

Skin-to-skin contact is crucial if you want your baby to return to the breast. Let your baby put on only diapers during breastfeeding attempts. Nurse him without a shirt and bra. A baby carrier or sling can help keep your baby close to you between breastfeeding attempts. Feeling your bare skin will soothe him. Also, try to nurse him when in a warm bath together. You can even allow him to sleep near you.

263

You may get your baby to nurse if you try when he is sleepy. Try breastfeeding him when he isn't fully awake or about to sleep.

Try nursing while in motion. Walking or rocking your baby may calm him and encourage him to nurse.

Changing your nursing position may also help. It will enable you to find out the position that is comfortable for your baby. Your baby is likely to nurse if he is relaxed during feeding.

Try nursing your baby frequently. Manipulating the breast to stimulate letdown before attempting breastfeeding can be helpful. Besides, you can use a dropper to drip expressed milk into his mouth when you attempt nursing him. Getting the milk without sucking for some seconds before letdown may encourage him to nurse.

A baby who refuses to breastfeed after previously doing so may not be weaning himself especially if he is under a year. However, the refusal to nurse may be due to infection, reaction to stress, new pregnancy or other conditions. The above tips can also be helpful when encouraging a fussy baby to breastfeed. In both cases, you have to be patient and persistently encourage your baby to nurse.

Getting your baby back to breast requires time. Try nursing him frequently. Coax him to latch on the breast. However, give him a break if he becomes upset during attempted breastfeeding. Forcing him to take the breast when he is frustrated will only make him have negative feelings towards nursing.

Also, try to maintain your milk supply by manually expressing or pumping your breast. You can feed your baby the expressed milk during the nursing strike. You can also drip the milk into his mouth when you attempt nursing him. Be persistent; your baby will get back to his breastfeeding routine with time.

CHAPTER 17

INVERTED NIPPLES

The indentation of nipples is a common breast variation. It can occur in both men and women. It may develop during childhood, puberty or even after surgery. Some women who don't have inverted nipples may experience this condition during pregnancy, especially if it is their first pregnancy.

In some cases, though rare, nipple inversion can be associated with trauma, breast cancer, infection such as mastitis, and abscess formation. You need to see a doctor if any or both of your nipples begin to turn inwards when you aren't pregnant or didn't have breast surgery.

The degree of inversion varies. It is temporary if it can be reversed by stimulation or changes in temperature. However, these methods cannot make permanently inverted nipples to become erect. There are other techniques that can make such nipples to protrude. You may experience different levels of inversion in each of your nipples or just in one nipple.

Are your nipples inverted?

Your nipples are retracted or flat if they aren't erect or don't protrude. Instead of pointing out, such nipples move inwards or retract into the breast tissue. The indentation may look like a dimple or a slit at the tip of the breast. A "pinch test" will help you determine whether you have an inverted nipple. Perform this test on both breasts.

Firmly place your areola between your thumb and index finger. Then, gently press about an inch into the breast. A normal nipple stays protruded while an inverted one retracts or flattens. The degree of inversion of nipples varies. You can pull out a slightly inverted nipple with your fingers. However, a nipple may appear as a dimple when it deeply retracts into the areola.

The indentation doesn't interfere with nipple sensitivity. Though it has no negative impact on your health, it may pose a challenge to breastfeeding. An inverted nipple that remains erect when pulled out doesn't cause any problem during nursing. However, nipples that tend to retract after being pulled out or those that cannot be pulled out make breastfeeding difficult or impossible.

Dealing with inverted nipples

Inverted nipples may cause your baby to struggle with latching. However, many women with retracted nipples can successfully breastfeed. Some techniques can help pull your nipples out if the inversion interferes with breastfeeding.

Hoffman method: A manual self-manipulation of the nipples with your hands can help bring them out. However, the effect of this stimulation approach may not last long. You need to regularly practice this technique (at least once daily) to make your nipples stand erect more often.

With your thumbs placed on each side of the base of your nipple, firmly press into the breast tissue. Gently move your thumbs around the nipple and away from each other while still pressing the tissue. Repeat the process severally to draw out the nipple. However, the Hoffman technique may not work for some nursing mothers with inverted nipples. The period the nipples will remain erect also differs among individuals.

Use of breast shells: These are plastic discs worn over the breast and inside the bra to draw out the nipples. You can use them between feeds. However, they can contribute to nipple confusion.

Nipple shields: They can help your baby to grasp the nipples. This device is a flexible and thin nipple-shaped silicone with holes at the tips. You can use a nipple shield to pull out the nipple during feedings. The breast milk reaches the baby through the openings at the tip of the device. However, incorrect use of the shield may frustrate the baby.

Suction devices such as cups, shells, nipple shields or extractors can make the nipples protrude for longer periods. These devices are worn on the breast and inside the bras. They loosen the nipple tissue and stimulate the nipples, making them to stay erect. Seek the advice of a lactation consultant before using any

273

of these devices to avoid further nursing problems.

Manual stimulation can make the nipples to be temporarily erect but nipple piercing and surgery can give lasting results. However, you should be aware of the risks associated with these options if you may want to breastfeed in future. Some surgeries can stop milk production while piercing may slow down your ability to nurse a baby.

Breastfeeding with inverted nipples

Babies are likely to experience difficulties compressing the milk ducts in severe cases of inversion. Despite the degree of inversion, you can breastfeed your baby. You need the help of a lactation consultant to establish a good latch. However, the presence of other latching problems such as a tongue tie can make breastfeeding difficult if you have inverted nipples.

In some cases, retracted nipples may not interfere with breastfeeding. Your baby can still nurse if he successfully takes the areola into his mouth. Though rare, this nursing problem may lead to constant sore nipples. This painful condition results when your baby compresses the retracted nipples instead of the milk ducts. Consequently, the infant will not obtain much milk.

Natural remedies may not be effective in all cases of nipple inversion. Besides, piercing and surgery have clear cut drawbacks that can affect breastfeeding. Despite the challenge posed by inverted nipples to nursing mothers, you can still nurse your baby. The following tips can help if you find it difficult to breastfeed with inverted nipples.

Use of breast pump: You can stimulate milk flow with a pump before you put your baby to the breast. If your baby still finds it difficult to make a good latch when the milk has started flowing, use nipple shields.

Nipple stimulation before feedings: Manipulate your nipple with your fingers. Move it between your index finger and thumb for a couple of minutes. Then, gently massage it with a wet and cold cloth for some seconds. However, you need to be careful to prevent your nipple from becoming numb due to the cold treatment. Lack of sensation can slow-down your letdown reflex.

Pull back the breast tissue: With all your fingers placed at the base of your nipple, push the breast tissue backward before your baby latches. This action will stimulate milk flow and cause the nipple to protrude.

A proper latch will also help. Assist your baby to make a deep latch by taking a good portion of the breast into his mouth and not just the nipple. Make sure he opens his mouth wide as he latches. It will enable him to take the entire areola into his mouth. (Guide on making a good latch is on Chapter 4)

Breastfeeding can be difficult for some moms with inverted nipples. However, the tips given above can help. Also, you can seek the assistance of a lactation consultant.